PRESBYOPIA

Therapies and Further Prospects

PRESBYOPIA
Therapies and Further Prospects

Alain-Nicolas Gilg MD

Medical Director
Lyon's Wilson Eye Center
Lyon, France

Foreword

Hullo Alain

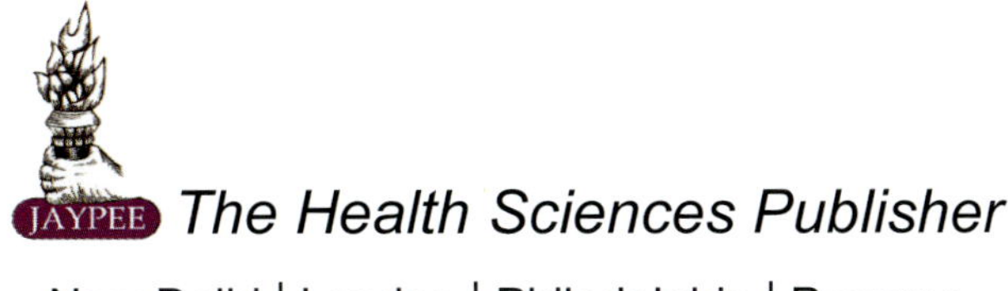

The Health Sciences Publisher

New Delhi | London | Philadelphia | Panama

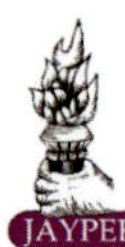 **Jaypee Brothers Medical Publishers (P) Ltd.**

Headquarters

Jaypee Brothers Medical Publishers (P) Ltd.
4838/24, Ansari Road, Daryaganj
New Delhi 110 002, India
Phone: +91-11-43574357
Fax: +91-11-43574314
E-mail: jaypee@jaypeebrothers.com

Overseas Offices

J.P. Medical Ltd.
83, Victoria Street, London
SW1H 0HW (UK)
Phone: +44 20 3170 8910
Fax: +44 (0)20 3008 6180
E-mail: info@jpmedpub.com

Jaypee-Highlights Medical Publishers Inc.
City of Knowledge, Bld. 237, Clayton
Panama City, Panama
Phone: +1 507-301-0496
Fax: +1 507-301-0499
E-mail: cservice@jphmedical.com

Jaypee Medical Inc.
The Bourse
111, South Independence Mall East
Suite 835, Philadelphia, PA 19106, USA
Phone: +1 267-519-9789
E-mail: jpmed.us@gmail.com

Jaypee Brothers Medical Publishers (P) Ltd.
17/1-B, Babar Road, Block-B, Shaymali
Mohammadpur, Dhaka-1207
Bangladesh
Mobile: +08801912003485
E-mail: jaypeedhaka@gmail.com

Jaypee Brothers Medical Publishers (P) Ltd.
Bhotahity, Kathmandu, Nepal
Phone: +977-9741283608
E-mail: kathmandu@jaypeebrothers.com

Website: www.jaypeebrothers.com
Website: www.jaypeedigital.com

© 2015, Jaypee Brothers Medical Publishers

Inquiries for bulk sales may be solicited at: jaypee@jaypeebrothers.com

Presbyopia: Therapies and Further Prospects

First Edition: 2015

ISBN: 978-93-5152-498-4

Printed at: Ajanta Offset & Packagings Ltd., New Delhi

Dedicated to

My daughters — Emeline and Maëlys

Foreword

Doctor Alain-Nicolas Gilg's work will interest all who read it, and with good reason. Dr Gilg writes passionately about the well-known condition of presbyopia and the methods for treating it. He covers this complicated subject using scientific language mixed with common terms so that it can be easily understood. He combines clearly written explanations with well-rendered illustrations. The book will be very useful, notably for future ophthalmologists, as it gives clear advice on the use of specific tests, such as refractive measurement in children and the refractive examination of patients with hyperopia.

Dr Gilg deals with various topics regarding accommodation and its mechanisms. He discusses the relationship between presbyopia and the different ametropias (hyperopia, myopia), as well as the possible optical compensations with correcting glasses, with the so-called progressive lenses or orthokeratological contact lenses.

Firstly, he defines accommodation, the eye's extraordinary ability to increase its power of convergence. Convergence, simply stated, is the ocular ability to focus light falling from a given distance to a single plane on the retina, by modifying the curvature of the lens. Thus, objects at a finite distance are clearly focused on retina and therefore clearly seen. Crystalline lens covers more on his anterior face during accommodation. During the contraction of ciliary muscle, suspensory ligament relaxes and modifies crystalline lens shape. Accommodation responds to nervous regulation.

Secondly, presbyopia is put back in its scientific context. It appears to occur as a result of several connected ocular phenomena rather than a single causal mechanism. These include an increase in crystalline lens sphericity, anterior translation of the lens, the surrounding action of the iris and cerebral plasticity. Crystalline lens becomes rounder during accommodation; its equatorial diameter decreases and keeps growing in its anterior part (with the reduction of the distance between lens and ciliary muscle). Presbyopia is the loss in amplitude of accommodation. It will physiologically grow weaker as the subject ages, primarily because the lens capsule progressively loses elasticity throughout life. The *punctum proximum* (the nearest point, the eye can see clearly with maximum accommodation) moves backwards and is located beyond the usual distance of near vision (13 inches). This forces the viewer to move the viewed object farther away in order to place it in clear focus. Presbyopia affects everyone, but first symptoms typically appear around the age 42 to 45 years old for emmetropes (earlier for hyperopes), depending on the habits of each individual.

Finally, Dr Gilg moves on to cover the highly controversial surgical possibilities for correcting presbyopia. These surgical options use techniques based upon the concepts of monovision and multifocality. They include multifocal presby-LASIK, monovision LASIK, pre-lens implants, multifocal implants, intrastromal corneal ring segments (ICRS), ciliary body sclerotomies, scleral expansion bands and conductive keratoplasty.

In the book, the physician shares his experience, along with his development of a ciliozonular tension ring system, aimed at ensuring the tension of zonular fibers, among other things.

There are many techniques having the goal of restoring accommodation. However, only the test of time, as well as the scientific certification of one or more of these techniques, will allow suggesting them to the patients with maximum safety. Whatever the technique used, it seems that it will be complemented with the classic solution of spectacles, whether fitted with ordinary single focus or progressive multifocal lenses.

Hullo Alain MD

Former Head of Ophthalmology
Department in Lyon-Sud Hospital, Lyon, France

Private Practice at Wilson Eye Center, Lyon, France, in Strabology and
Anterior Segment Surgery Department

Preface

God invented and gave us sight to the end that we might behold the courses of intelligence in the heaven, and apply them to the courses of our own intelligence.
— **Plato, Timaeus**

This book, aimed at well-informed readers, is above all a didactic and thorough treatment of the subject of presbyopia. Indeed, despite its complex theme, it still raises numerous questions from our patients and our friends. I voluntarily decided to present this arduous topic, in the same way, I would inform either a patient during a consultation, or our young medical students in the operating theater. Furthermore, this work is equally intended for the friends and family of our patients willing to update their knowledge of presbyopia. It is true that today, our refractive patients and these students look alike. In spite of often having insufficient pre-requisite or, even more regrettable, inaccurate or commonplace ideas, they have a great need for accurate information.

Our current role as ophthalmologists, at the risk of becoming technical advisors, is thus also to inform. Indeed, information is at the heart of the doctor-patient relationship, and this is for the best. Those days when ophthalmologists chose the most appropriate treatment, usually without possible or even wanted dialogue, are definitely past.

It is not uncommon in our ophthalmological clinical practice to examine a patient, who arrives apparently perfectly aware of what diagnostic gears to use, and the resulting potential diagnoses. The patient often knows the spontaneous or treated prognosis, has a good knowledge of the various possible treatments, and sometimes even treatments still in experimental stage! This is our daily routine.

As a matter of fact, in order to relieve, compensate and treat our patients' refractive problems, it is part of our duty to know all the therapeutic means at our disposal.

The level of detail provided by current methods enables us to give clear, fair information and to carry out actions. This is done in accordance with the most recently updated scientific information, as they are defined by the code of medical ethics. It is a matter of determining the best treatment strategy for the patients according to their wishes. They are then able to make the most of their corrected eyesight, and will effortlessly take advantage of a full range of vision, distance, intermediate or near, at different levels of brightness. It is about strategy because, as we will see, the modification of a visual factor can lead to the evolution of other visual variables.

This technical and technological environment, in aid of the patients, finds itself in ophthalmologic offices or centers and, as a result, the practitioner's investment, in terms of continuing education and financial effort, is significant. Our patients, expecting high-performance, quick and optimized surgery, must be ready to afford high fares and accept low repayments.

The notified reader will gain, page after page, the necessary elements to comprehend the accommodative phenomena stemming from the diverse troubles of vision. He or she should by then, be better armed to understand what functional influences the eruption of presbyopia has over the world's grandma-boomer population.

Given the colossal figures it represents, presbyopia is undeniably a world ailment. Posing a real public health problem, in terms of prevalence and incidence, it also has major economic repercussions and considerable commercial stakes on the planet scale. In France, 27 million are presbyope, 19 million of whom are aged between 45 and 70, as officially listed in the year 2007. Presbyopia has got at 90 million of European individuals, almost as many North Americans, and more than 2 billion human beings on earth! What amazing figures: the reader should find enough motivation to carry on the book, insofar as he or she gets in medical and scientific literature beforehand, to familiarize with the related vocabulary.

We have made up our mind to get the reader to enter the reasoning sphere of modern ophthalmology and its medical jargon, its deductive approach and its critical analysis of present time therapeutics. Regarding the semantic difficulties, just as the scientific or medical gaps, the non-specialist reader might meet with, I have worked out a numbered cross-references from the text. In "Notes" chapter, you will find each uncleared notion mentioned in the book, as long as the digression does not take us too far away from our subject, and the explanation seems indispensable for the debate.

It is difficult to enter a closed world such as ophthalmology without first absorbing its language. It may well be the reason why our colleagues, who practice in different domains, consider us as specialists of our own.

What a shame, it would be for the reader to leave the track before the end of the introductory course! Besides, the search prospects are unexpected and, in near future, the development will bring a visual rejuvenation cure to who wants to get his youthful vision back.

I do hope the book will answer all the readers' questions, or at the very least, that it will provide them with elements likely to rouse their curiosity. As for those who think ocular-lift is no longer a wild dream, visionary researchers are at the right place.

Alain-Nicolas Gilg

Contents

CHAPTER 1

Accommodation and Presbyopia

1.1 DEFINITIONS AND SYMPTOMATOLOGY

In my ophthalmological practice, I do not spend a single day without dealing with a problem of my patients' presbyopia.

1.1.1 Etymologies

Also called presbytia, eyesight of the presbyope as presbyteros (πρεσβύτερος, the aging subject): it is the loss of the eye's accommodative power.

This definition of presbyopia does not prejudge the origin of the accommodative loss (traumatic, infectious, tumoral), the senile dysfunction (dystrophia) being the most frequent cause in its broadest acceptance: presbyopia.

Accommodation is the means by which the eye modifies its optical power in order to keep a sharp image on the retina (Fig. 1.1).

Its Latin origin (accommodātĭo, ōnis, f.) translates the action of adapting, adjusting, sorting out. It is indeed evoking, here, the idea of a dynamic focus of the vision while adapting to different distances, going from distant vision to near one, or the other way round.

Accommodation is a symmetrical and consensual phenomenon: that is to say, the ocular couple should accommodate the same value at the same time.

This consideration has its importance given that some patients present a problem of refraction that can disturb both eyes' simultaneous focus capacity, and then impair the quality of binocular fusion.

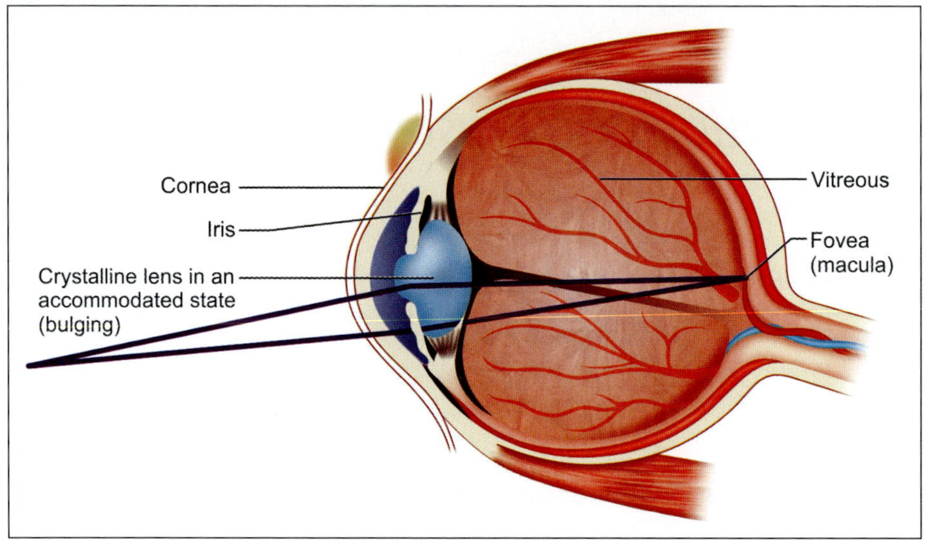

Fig. 1.1 Accommodating eye in a non-presbyopic patient

On a non-presbyopic eye, with straight gaze fixing, the focus works in central vision. Then, the image of a near object crosses the optical systems which focus it on the central foveal retina.

Binocular vision defines itself by its three grades:
- Grade I is the simultaneous vision or biocularity, this is the capacity to see double in binocular vision;
- Grade II is the fusion or binocularity, this is the capacity to see simple in binocular vision;
- Grade III is the stereoscopic vision or stereocularity; this is the capacity to see in binocular relief.

After these inescapable definitions, what are the symptoms of presbyopia?

1.1.2 Functional Signs

The functional signs are mainly the discomforts felt and mentioned by the patient, such as:
- blurred near vision,
- reading unusual fatigue,

- slow focus,
- headaches,
- tendency to hold reading at arm's length (the patients commonly say they need a "forearm graft"!),
- search for better lighting (to improve contrasts), or lack of interest in reading small capitals.

Many presbyopes rightly complain about the little consideration given to their "handicap":
- the use of small capitals (insurance contracts, drugs precautions),
- the poor quality of some printed documents,
- the overuse of colored texts on colored backgrounds, considerably reducing contrasts,
- and finally the bad quality of paper, whether recycled or not, spoiling the albedo of the page, as much as its legibility.

1.1.3 Physical Signs

Presbyopia also appears through physical signs, according to the patient, and confirmed by ocular redness after prolonged reading and lacrimations after near vision efforts.

Presbyopia does appear in some human activities. In pictorial art, the modification of the artists' sight can have more or less obvious consequences on their work. Let's take Rembrandt (1606–1669) as an example. We do not know anything about his ophthalmological condition, but the maturity of his work coincides with the introduction of impasto, a technique used in painting, where paint is laid very thickly with brush or painting-knife, usually thickly enough that the wide and vigorous strokes are visible. On none of his self-portraits does the Dutch painter represent correcting lenses or pince-nez. Since impasto does not demand a vision of details from the artist, this process is more typical of presbyopic artists whose first works do not contain any (last Titian's paintings). The optical explanation thus seems more plausible than the stylistic justification, although, judging by the handrest, the working distance of oil paint must have been stretched-arm distance, for this technique.

This being said, in accordance with its definition, presbyopia does not exist before the age of 38 years old. In case of an organic lesion, or accommodative asthenopia in purely functional situations, it is then called presbyopia.

The whole symptomatology shares aspects allowing some diagnosis: the disorders concern both eyes at the same time, start around forty, then get to expand with no possible regression, except at the beginning of the affection.

Because it is an age-related affection, as opposed to a "disease", what I tend to repeat to patients concerned, not to say depressed while they face unexpected handicap.

1.2 PREVALENCE AND INCIDENCE OF PRESBYOPIA

Neither in the human race, nor amongst the superior primates, there is no one who escapes it; except for some of the patients who do not follow the usual development of presbyopia, for reasons that have still to be figured out.

1.2.1 Compared Ontogeny

As Professor Pouliquen[1] emphasizes it, it is interesting to notice that in the animal species adventure of eye's development, the mammals keep an ontological memory of their aquatic origin.

Consequently, during the accommodation, the human race uses the advantages of:
- stenopeisation (Cephalopod's eye),
- focal dynamic (Copilia's visual system),
- biotopical ametropization (Aquatrols' visual organ).

All the unavoidability, bilaterality and symmetry of the presbyopia phenomenon plead in favor of a still widely discussed dynamic process of tissular aging.

From a finalist viewpoint, it is interesting to notice how nature has endowed the human beings with accommodative power decreasing during life.

1.2.2 Various Enlarger Systems in Vertebrates

In vertebrates, many systems permit to enlarge the images.

We notice a power increase in corneal diopter during the air quest (reptiles, birds, mammals), crystalline movements when it is spherical and not deformable (abyssal fish) and finally possible deformations (birds and mammals).

Fish eye is big and made of a scleral shell, particularly developed in deep sea species, allowing a resistance to pressure. A flat cornea and a great crystalline lens not deformable and spherical are typical of this eye.

Fishes are going to accommodate to see in the distance by moving their crystalline lenses backwards towards the retina thanks to a muscle (Figs 1.2A and B).

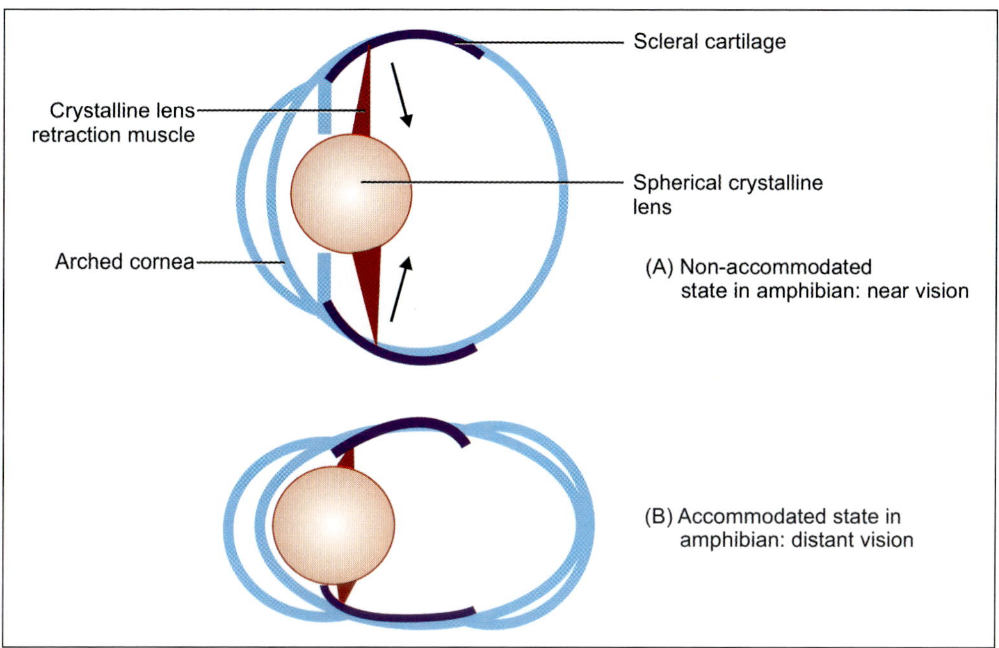

Figs 1.2A and B Accommodation in fish. Paradoxically, and because of the aquatic environment refractive index, the fish accommodates (B) to see in the distance and rests in near vision (A)

During the amphibians (Figs 1.3A and B) and reptiles (Figs 1.4A and B) air quest, lacrymal glands as well as eyelids allow cornea hydration modifying curvature radius to adapt to refraction index change between outdoor (air) and indoor (water) but accommodation occurs just as for fish, with crystalline lens moving.

In mammals, crystalline lens takes a lenticular shape and can deform itself thanks to a complex muscular system.

The most advanced system belongs to the diving/fishing birds such as the cormorant where the very large eye occupies the whole eye-socket.

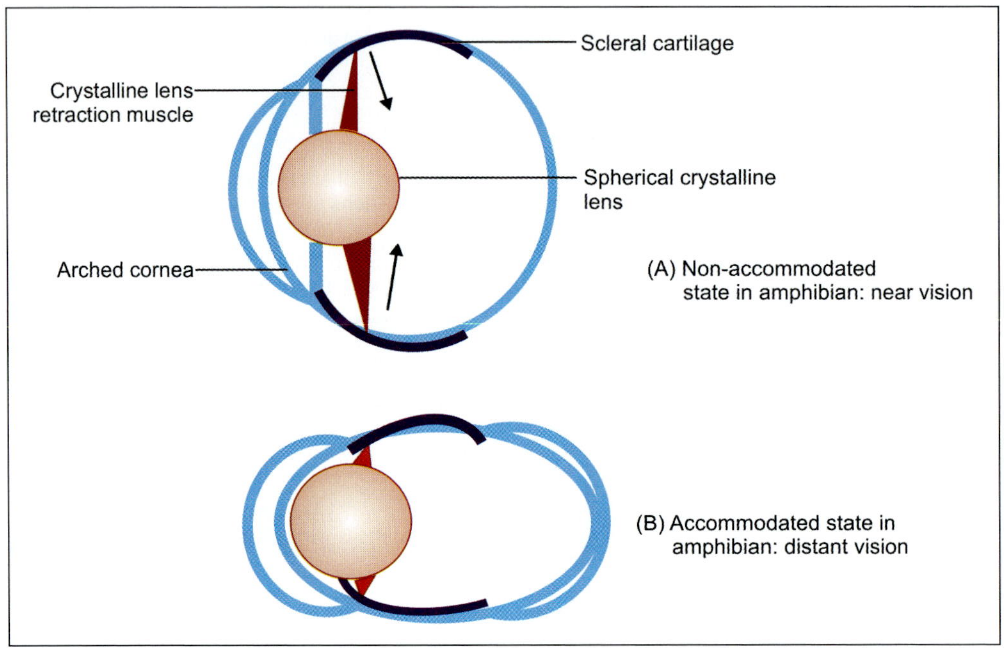

Figs 1.3A and B Accommodation in amphibian. From their aquatic origins, like fish the amphibians accommodate for distant vision (B) with the intervention of crystalline lens retraction muscle (A)

When the bird is diving, the Crompton muscle (Fig. 1.5A) allows the corneal flattening (like for fish), and under the action of Brüch's muscle, crystalline lens can deform until forming a lenticonus (Fig. 1.5B).

The cormorant can thus have optical power vary from around 50 diopters!

Great sea predators, sharks for instance, do not base their hunter capacities upon visual sense. Effectively, high myopes, sharks compensate deficient vision with hearing, sense of smell, of touch and above all electromagnetism (pores, ampullae of Lorenzini, located on the surface of the body) to detect their prey or spot the possible coming of enemies. Hammerhead sharks have their eyes at the end of the two cephalic extensions.

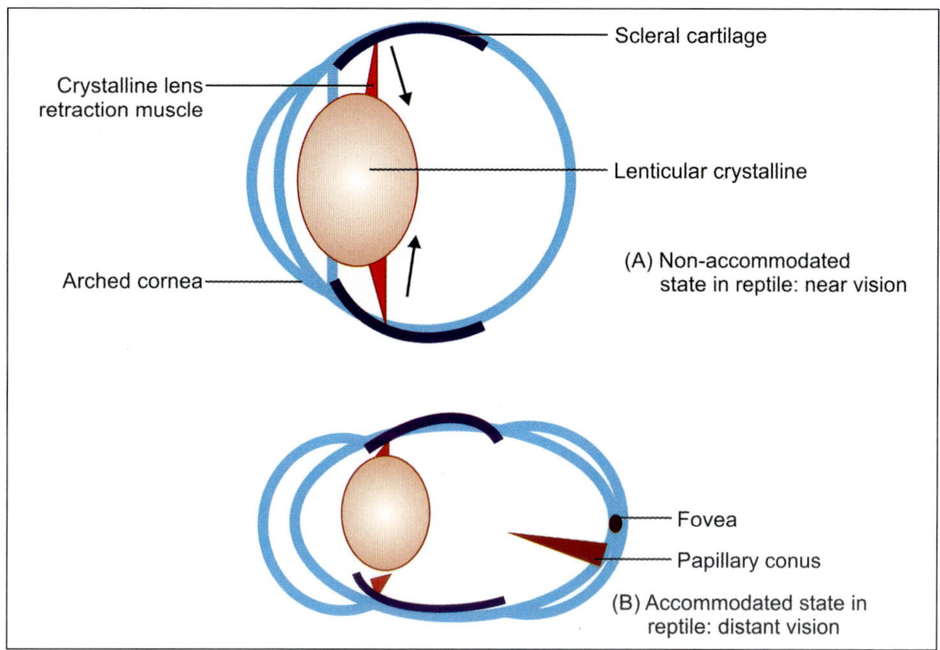

Figs 1.4A and B Accommodation in reptiles. Like in fish (where they come from) and the amphibians, reptiles accommodate to see in the distance by contracting the crystalline lens retraction muscle (A). Crystalline lens lenticular shape seems to be an adaptation to life on earth. Lizards have a fovea and reptiles have a vitreous less liquefied than fish and amphibians with persisting papillary conus, a vitreous vestigial vascularization (B)

Sharks' voluminous eyes are mobile thanks to the intervention of some muscles. They also have two thick and still eyelids to protect them. In some shark species, there is a winking membrane considered as a third transversal and mobile eyelid. It serves as a protection by covering the eye while the shark is about to bite. The transparent cornea is flattened and prolonged with an extremely resistant sclerotic, partly cartilaginous. The protruding crystalline lens is almost spherical: exaggerated convexity, added to the fact it does not deform itself much or easily accommodate, explains the shark myopia. According to the species, the pupil is often round or oval. Apart from this quasi-non-existent accommodation, sharks see colors, contrasts,

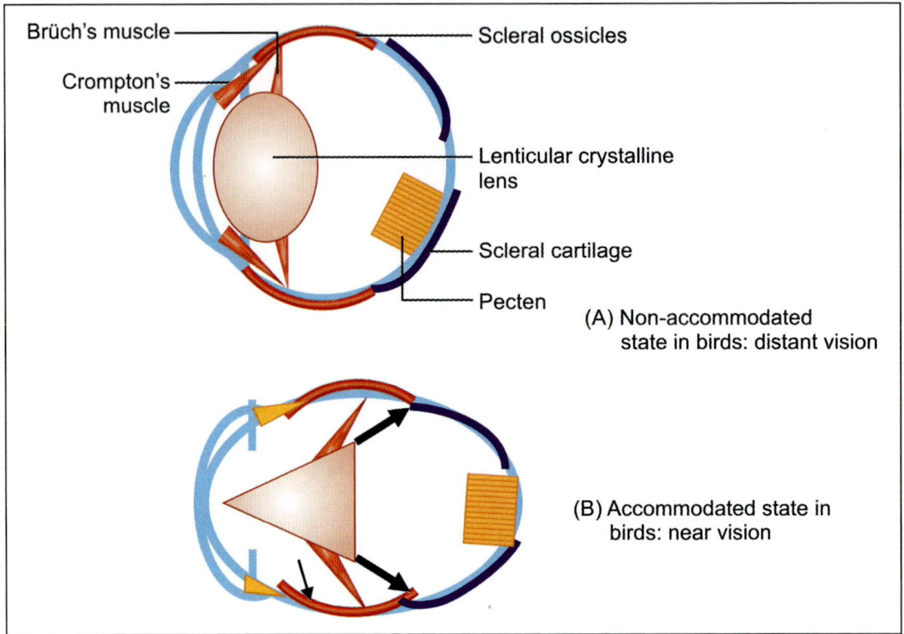

Figs 1.5A and B Accommodation in birds. The bird's eye looks like the mammals' one insofar as the accommodated state enables near vision thanks to muscles deforming crystalline lens and cornea leaning on a sclera's hard part (cartilage, ossicles) (A). The bird's accommodated eye then takes the shape of "a bell" (B)

regulate the sudden variations in surrounding light intensity (bright tapestry or tapetum lucidum), have a high sensitivity as opposed to a low visual acuity.

Myopes, presbyopes, astigmats and animals also affected by natural cataract: it seems that nature has not been really kind to bovines.

Having a protruding crystalline lens, bovines own a near vision enabling them to see herb in front of them very clearly (Fig. 1.6). However, on the contrary, since ciliary muscles are not worked out, accommodation capacity remains quite low for distant vision.

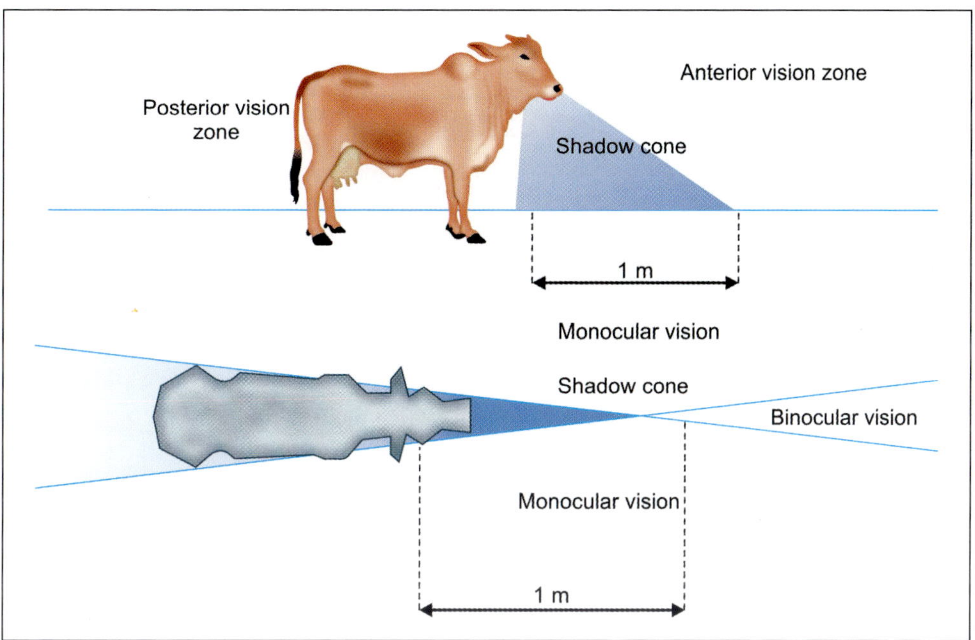

Fig. 1.6 Bovine vision

1.2.3 Accommodative Involution

So the infant's mother, while holding him in her arms and instinctively coming closer, until standing only few centimeters from him, thus provides him with the capacity of a 20 diopters near accommodation, meaning clear vision until 5 cm for an emmetropic subject, just as the distance between him and the rattle in his hand.

An emmetropic eye is an eye that does not show any refractive disorders. When accommodation is not processing, this eye sees a far-off object: focus is on the retina (Fig. 1.7).

As child grows up, accommodative power progressively decreases and seems to match visual needs. It happens at the time of walk, draw learning, and while developing fine motricity. So many parents tell me,

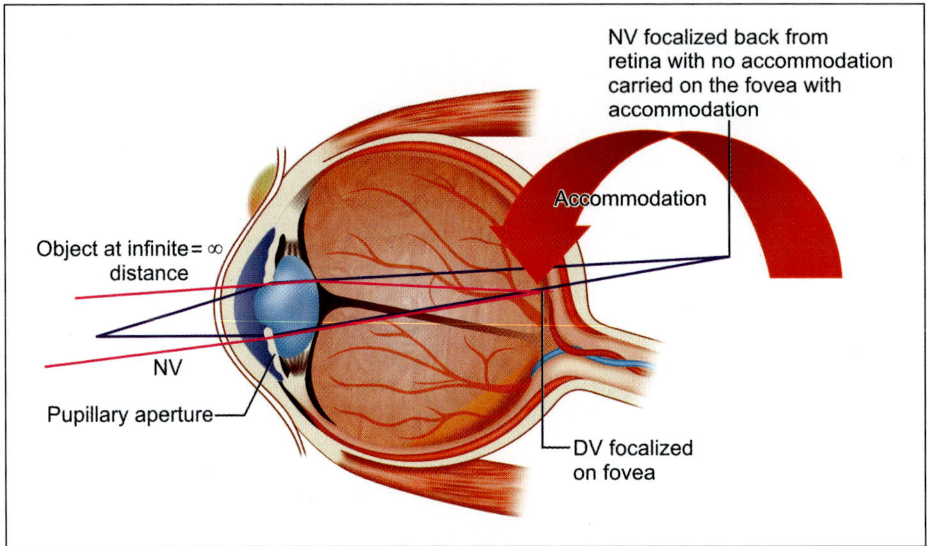

Fig. 1.7 Distant, near vision and accommodation in a non-presbyopic not compensated emmetrope

In emmetropes, an image located to infinite (DV = Distant Vision: in practice, more than 5 meters) crosses the pupillary aperture and the eye's transparent media. It then converges on the fovea (no accommodation). As for a near object (NV = Near Vision), the emmetropic eye passively focuses at the back of the retina, but the accommodation allows an active focus on the fovea.

"Doctor, you are saying my baby may well need spectacles, and yet, he is able to find a minute thread hidden in the fitted-carpet."

In the absence of other refractive problems, physiological accommodative loss progressively leads to keep only a residual accommodation diopter. It occurs without bothering the subject during his first 40 years, until 60 years old.

At 60, the accommodative capacity of the lens would be nil. Nonetheless, the ocular globe's plasticity allows it to keep a field depth of 1.00 diopter. In addition, we observe this phenomenon on patients who had their lens removed (aphakia).

The decrease of the so-called accommodation amplitude, that is to say the values range, expressed in diopters (by analogy to prismatic diopters deflecting light), is not a time-related linear function.

Nevertheless, certain practitioners refer to some empirical table of the age expected addition (Table 1.1).

Addition is the dioptrical power attributed to glasses part allotted to near vision. The value of this addition added with the prescription of the distant vision, gives the compensatory power value in near vision, together with a sharp and comfortable vision.

Table 1.1 Expected addition (expressed in diopters) according to the patient's age, for a working distance of 40 cm

Addition	+0.50	+0.75	+1.00	+1.25	+1.50	+1.75	+2.00	+2.25	+2.50
Age	40	42	44	46	48	50	52	56	60

The complexity of the system has a variable speed of deterioration, based upon biological non-unitarian factors laid out in series. It follows a biomechanical exhaustion, which we would rather qualify as viscoelastical, if we could establish a biophysical modelization.

Contrary to other affections in medicine, presbyopia does not present any gender or race's characteristic. Its prevalence and incidence are identical for men and women, for Caucasians, Asians, or melanoderms.

Environmental factors themselves do not seem to play a major role in this affection, whether they are biotope's latitude grade, sunlight, diet habits, life socioeconomical conditions, or ergonomy at workstation. Even in unilateral or bilateral amblyopia (defect in functional development of the vision with no anatomical impairment).

Statistically, none of these elements seems to influence the emergence of this affection within the population. So, as far as accommodation is concerned, would our organism, remarkable system, then be destined to a genetically programmed involution like a species' characteristic?

It is far from being certain. At a time when molecular genetics is proudly cited in the media, when geneticians and biologists solve more enigma of human genome every day, nobody has yet discovered a series of genes commanding accommodation and presbyopia.

Even so, searchers identify genes that accelerate ocular aging in glaucoma, macular degeneration bound to the age, pigmentary degeneration of the retina and the other familial heredomacular degenerations.

Nothing seems to hamper the inescapable way to presbyopia, but nothing can accelerate it either, except pharmacological actions. We will come back to this later (*See* paragraph 1.3.3, Convergence, page 14).

Sleep deprivation or jetlag, usually faced in critical situations, in emergency medicine, or aeronautical medicine, are ordeals intensely felt by the organism, which sets adaptations for the various organs of relation life. If the threshold of vigilance lessens, along with the fall of its attendant superior brain function, the other vital functions, pulmonary and cardiac ones, remain untouched, just as the other vegetative functions, especially digestive and urinary ones. It is as if the organism in difficulty centered its adaptation efforts on elements essential to survival. This is also the case of the situations of great malnutrition due to starvation or hunger strike.

In all these extreme situations, accommodation and the ongoing presbyopia seem preserved, what tends to link intrinsic processes to vegetative functions, normally unconscious and involuntary.

There does not seem to be any hormonal influence over accommodation or the course of presbyopia: pregnant woman and endocrine diseased people, apart from secondary cataracts they may have, do not suffer from either accommodation problems or premature presbyopia. Nonetheless, some medical books typically confirm a quicker development of presbyopia in the presence of certain affections: open angle glaucoma, diabetes, myasthenia, Graves' disease, debilitating affections, overwork, and neurosis.[2]

1.3 ANATOMICAL PATHWAYS OF ACCOMMODATION

Accommodation and presbyopia thus represent quite a singular entity in the organism and its physiological processes. Neurological pathways of accommodation are in close relation with oculomotricity pathways and pupillary motility.

In usual situation, the frontal motor areas voluntarily activate the accommodation at the cerebral cortex level. They give this order to the brain stem's motor nucleus by a descending pathway.

The stimulation of both Perlia and Edinger-Westphals' nucleus provokes, on a healthy subject, the activation of three simultaneous, indissociable in time and in space, joint actions: it is about the synkinetic reflex of accommodation-miosis convergence.

1.3.1 Synkinesis

This is the phenomenon implemented to read this book in near vision. The ocular couple puts itself in convergence, meaning in oculomuscular adduction, under the influence of the medial rectus muscle, stimulated by the oculomotor nerves. The convergence phenomenon happens at the same time as the accommodative focusing on the text along with the pupillary miosis. Pupils are stimulated in miosis by stimulation of the parasympathetic nervous contingent on its way to the iris annular sphincter constrictor muscle.

The corollary of this physiological observation is that the effect of the eye's extrinsic musculature, or pupillary motility, can indirectly activate the accommodation whether positively or negatively.

There are pharmacological or optical situations in which such interferences between accommodation, oculomotricity and pupillary mobility, are possible. Let us first view the old drugs, known since antiquity for their action on pupillary size.

1.3.2 Miosis

It is above all pilocarpine, an alkaloid molecule obtained from the leaves of tropical American shrubs called jaborandi. Thanks to its hydrophilic nature, its chlorhydrate formula, instilled on the surface of the eye, gets into the tissues and stimulates the iris sphincter's muscarinic receptor M3, thus provoking both miosis and ciliary spasm responsible for transitory spastic accommodation.

Conversely, atropine or its derivatives, belladonna extracts, acts with sulphated formula laid on the eye in instillation, by provoking pupillary dilation (mydriasis), together with cycloplegia (pharmacologically-induced paralysis of ciliary muscle).

Senescence ordinarily comes with a physiological decrease of the pupillary diameter which can somewhat bind the synkinetic reflex analysis.

The pupillary diameter in the population varies from 8.5 mm to 3.0 mm with a predominance of subjects between 5.5 and 4.5 mm.

Pupil, playing the role of an optical diaphragm, allows reducing some visual aberrations, the way a stenopeic hole placed before the eye would do it.

A stenopeic hole or pinhole camera is a mask with a hole of 1 mm pierced in the middle.

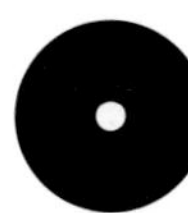

From this hole, light beam faces interference on the edge of the whole (pupillary bank) with increase in the image clearness (sensitivity to contrasts) and in the field depth (clear area on both sides of the image), but decrease in its intensity (which needs an image enlightened enough). Stenopeisation during accommodation contributes to near vision focus, in as much as the read page remains well illuminated.

1.3.3 Convergence

Moreover, convergence and accommodation are tightly bound during the synkinetic reflex. Excessive accommodation for children can come together with convergent strabismus, completely reversible in its pure form, after adequate correction of the refraction.

Other accommodative disorders, such as accommodative spasm, can go with spasmodic esotropia (or convergent strabismus) added with convergence, sometimes replaced by insufficient convergence in decompensate cases.

The etiologies of bilateral spasms are linked to intoxications with:
- opium,
- morphine,
- aconitine,
- digitaline,
- arsenobenzol, sulphonamides,
- general parasympathomimetic drug (jaborandi, Calabar beans),
- muscarine (amanita muscaria),
- parathion,
- curare, and
- exceptionally brought up, methylene blue.

Some neurological diseases can be responsible in cases of:
- diphtheria,
- certain encephalitis,
- meningitis,
- tabetic crisis,
- periodic spasm during oculomotor nerve cyclic phenomenon, and
- chorea, exceptionally.

Other affections can trigger accommodative spasms such as helminthiasis (ascariasis, oxyuriasis), hypervitaminosis B1, electrocution or different types of tooth extraction.

In all those etiologies, the instillation of cyclopegic cancels the signs (including inconstant macropsia).
Macropsia: enlarged appearance of seen objects. Contrary : micropsia (see below).

1.3.4 Accommodative Insufficiencies

However, accommodative insufficiencies from reduction or removal of accommodation, apart from crystalline lens affections or presbyopia, as mentioned earlier, are most of the time related to ciliary muscle palsies.

These palsies settle suddenly, or sometimes, progressively, and might be associated with signs like inconstant micropsia (see above for definition), as well as frequent paralytic mydriasis stemming from the relations, previously described, between accommodation and pupil (*See* paragraph 1.3.1, Synkinesis, page 12).

Then light can remove the pupillary reflex while convergence preserves it, what the anatomical distinction of those two reflex chains emphasizes. This is Argyll Robertson's sign that associates a removal of the pupillary contraction by light and preservation of synkinetic miosis, with accommodation-convergence.

Conversely, during synkinetic accommodation-convergence of near vision with a preserved pupil light reflex, we also notice an abnormality of the pupillary contraction: this is the reverse Argyll Robertson's sign.

Both of them cover various etiologies: neurological, traumatic ones, intoxications and miscellaneous affections.

Eyeball traumas add areflexive mydriasis to cycloplegia as in the related case of hymenoptera stings to sclerocorneal limbus.

We can also observe cycloparesis in cranial trauma with third nerve paralysis or thoracic trauma, or even in case of electrocution.

Cycloparesis can occur with ocular pathologies such as subacute glaucoma, uveitis or congenital aniridia.

A few intoxications and the absorption of some products may lead to bilateral cycloplegia. Especially the use of certain anticholinergical active drugs, well known for their contraindication if there is a risk of glaucoma by iridocorneal angle closure:

- solanaceae species,
- belladonna and its derivatives (homatropine, tropicamide, cyclopentolate),
- scopolamine,
- antiparkinsonians,
- synthetic antihistaminics,

- ganglioplegics (hexamethonium, tetraethylammonium chloride),
- central nervous system stimulants, tranquillizers (chlorpromazine, phenothiazines),
- monkshood,
- anticoagulants,
- organic arsenicals,
- barbiturates,
- sodium and potassium bromides,
- allyl dibromide,
- carbon bisulfide,
- cannabis,
- carbon monoxide, carbon dioxide,
- chloral,
- chloramphenicol,
- chloroquine,
- cinchonine sulfate,
- coniine and conhydrine,
- dinitrophenol, disulphone,
- iodoform,
- Virginia jasmine,
- henbane, mecamylamine,
- mercury and its salts,
- diphenylhydantoine methyl,
- methyl bromide and chloride,
- nutmeg,
- hydrogen phosphide,
- morphine,
- estrogens, ponalide,
- quinine,
- sulfamides,
- sodium and potassium thioglycolates,
- valerian,

- valethamate bromide,
- lead,
- ergot,
- antidiphteric vaccine,
- food poisoning,
- poisonous fungus, and
- snake venom.

Some infections and parasitosis going with cycloplegia:
- leprosy,
- diphtheria,
- botulism,
- tetanus,
- dengue,
- epidemic hepatitis,
- trichinosis,
- ankylostomiasis, and
- amebiasis.

Neurological affections come with ciliary muscle palsy during the clinical affection of an internal ophthalmoplegia with third nerve lesion:
- Economo's disease (encephalitis lethargica),
- Infectious encephalitis (measles, mumps, typhoid fever, scarlet fever, cow pox, influenza, undetermined viruses),
- neuro-syphilis,
- tuberculous meningitis,
- Heine-Medin disease,
- Guillain-Barré syndrome (acute idiopathic polyneuritis),
- Little's disease,
- posterior cranial fossa syndrome, and
- Wilson's disease.

The appearance of bilateral cycloparesis has implied several metabolic and endocrine disorders:

- diabetes,
- Graves' disease,
- lactation,
- avitaminosis (B1, B2, C),
- depression, and
- anoxia.

Some lesions, close to the pathway of the oculomotor nerve, can breed a more or less important and more or less reversible palsy of the ciliary muscle. As it is the case in sphenoid sinusitis, dental affection, or other causes like Takayashu's disease, pithiatism or simulation.

That long and tedious list of what causes ciliary muscle palsy, which leads to some near-vision isolated affection, still shows the complexity of the ciliary effector accommodation pathway. It also proves that, in bilateral forms, the diversity of contexts can get us to diagnose a starting presbyopia, whereas it is a secondary loss of accommodation, which is often caused by:

- certain affections,
- unknown administration of anticholinergical drug,
- clinical forms of diphtheria, botulism, tetanus, encephalitis, syphilis, diabetes, brainstem or hypophyseal fossa tumor.

In the absence of ciliary muscle, the congenital forms show familial bilateral palsy, hereditary and of predominant autosomal genetic transmission.

As we will see this further (*See also* paragraph 2.2.1, Hyperopic compensation, page 47), hyperopia in its acquired form, and which, according to its value, requires uncomfortable accommodation to focus, also expresses itself throughout a near-vision isolated affection.

Oculo-orbital affections leading to unilateral hyperopia represent local causes: orbital tumor lying in the retrobulbar cone, an intraocular tumor concerning the posterior pole, idiopathic retinal detachment, retinal or secondary chorioretinal detachment, exudative suffusion, in the macular region, some retinal detachment surgeries (with reduction of the scleral surface), ocular hypotonia which may bring about axial hyperopia (such after glaucoma filtering surgeries); some scars, corneal flattening, whether traumatically-induced or not (superficial or deep keratitis after corneal wound healing).

Astigmatisms, we will come back to it (*See also* paragraph 2.4, Presbyopia and astigmatisms, page 60), can give simultaneous affection of near and distal vision.

Optical correction just cannot solve all lowering visions.

Affections ones we are interested in are mainly transient and they appear as some visual disorder when accommodation changes, what is known as accommodotonia.

This neologism goes to show a slowing down in the accommodated states changes. As mentioned before, not only is accommodotonia the main reason why the new presbyopes should consult, but it is also present in unbalanced diabetes, of chronic alcoholism, Graves' disease, cluster headache, some cases of cranial trauma, syphilis, measles, or in streptomycin historical treatment, obviously in connection with some neurological or selective muscular problem.

As for children, the accommodative fall or loss involving a difficulty or impossibility to read remains exceptional, no matter what the underlying refractive disorder may be, due to the high accommodative amplitude explained above. After a complete ophthalmic check-up along with pharmacological provocation test, it has to look after a brutal decompensation of unknown high ametropia, or a simulation (child's reactional depression to a divorce, after family loss, or other psychological trauma).

1.4 ACCOMMODATIVE OPTOMETRY

As it is often the case in medicine, all affection deserves a qualification, which is precisely what we have been considering until now (*See* paragraph 1.3.4, Accommodative insufficiencies, page 15).

Moreover, accommodation and presbyopia require quantitative assessment to determine the status of the affection, understand its functional slowing down, predict its evolution, and to appreciate therapeutic efficiency. Then how can we get a method to measure presbyopia?

1.4.1 Measures

In practice, not to disturb the synkinetic reflex (*See* paragraph 1.3.1, Synkinesis, page 12), we determine the accommodative power of both eyes in biocular vision, and we can carry out the examination in various luminance conditions (scotopic or nocturnal environment, mesopic or twilight intermediate one, photopic or diurnal surrounding).

Lighting conditions play no small part in it, for it determines how easily, quickly, precisely, and how amply the vision is able to adjust the focus thanks to the contrasts.

If we cannot have the reading light vary, we can also propose, in photopic conditions, to get optotypes varied in contrast (20%, 50%, 70%, 100% saturation), on a white background.

As we usually notice it in far visual acuity test type, for sociocultural reasons, numerical optotypes are an alternative to alphabetical optotypes (no Roman alphabet, pronunciation difficulties, schooling level).

Optotypes are the characters on the eye charts used to measure visual acuity.

However, all these optotypes of morphoscopic determination in visual acuity (alphanumerical optotypes, drawings, Snellen, "C" or Landolt's rings) have sensitivity different from the optotypes representing the visual acuity in network (sinusoidal stimuli) or the angular visual acuity (Landolt's ring), which we can use for near vision.

Some related periodicals propose a near visual acuity, expressed in percentage of central visual efficiency, where 100% is an excellent visual acuity.

Nevertheless, usual measuring systems did not obtain international recognition for the rating scale lacks linearity decimal visual acuity, textual content (revised standard Parinaud and Jaeger scale, American type point, notation "M"), possible interferences with the ametropias (dioptric scale).

Regarding its accuracy in high and low visions, we should only use the spatial resolution logMAR chart of the minimal angle, since the diversity of the normative pads excludes all possibility of getting used to it, or of interference with underlying ametropia, if any.

Immediate precisions to the reader about the fact that, in near vision, instead of using aim devices, we must favor the use of optotypes chart. Indeed, its stand is unfailing, its whiteness impeccable, the page albedo and reflectance are controlled.

1.4.2 Ergonomics

Effectively, the automatic refractor for the optometric consultations, as well as the screening visiotest used in occupational medicine, both have the faculty of leading, for a certain number of our patients, to an accommodation impairing the performance test whether in near, intermediate or distance vision.

The static measure of near vision, graded 40 cm (35 cm for others, 14 inches in the USA), only gives partial account of accommodative efforts necessary from far to near vision, through the intermediate one (an arm's length eye-to-computer screen distance).

We measure dynamic near vision by evaluation of the reading speed. It is quantified by the number of per-minute words the subject can read in a running text, supposing he or she has acquired the principles of reading and disposes of a normal visuospatial strategy (normal population read at a pace between 140 and 250 words/minute).

The recent revival of interest in posturology among visuomotor disorders (dyslexia, dysgraphia, visuospatial dyspraxia) allows to screen and take charge of proprioceptive deficiency syndromes causing various problems (exaggerated headache while reading, feeling to read without understanding). These syndromes of postural deficiency are frequent within the population, since we have estimated that 5 to 10% show dysproprioceptive symptomatology.

Not being as conspicuous as the sense of hearing, eyesight or smell, proprioception is an occult sense often forgotten by doctors and patients, despite concerning several organs. It is still essential for body tonico-postural regulation in time and space (somesthesia) (*See also* paragraph 3.1.3, Multifocal lenses, page 84). This is why its dysfunction hampers normal reading flow, adequate concentration and normal regulation of muscular contractility. It explains the exacerbation of signs we observe when presbyopia starts, for an adult who was not posturally reprogrammed during childhood (*See also* bibliography, "SDP et l'ophtalmologie autrement", page 204).

Accommodative course or amplitude gives the most elements about the accommodative capacities of the subject at a given time of the day, without considering fatigability factor.

1.4.3 Tests

1.4.3.1 Search for Maximal Accommodation

In practice, we advise the "push-up test" technique with a patient corrected in distance vision. This method consists of asking the patient to stare at the smallest visible text on reading board standing one meter from him, then to bring it closer and closer until the text gets illegible.

The distance covered (expressed in centimeter) gives the subject's accommodative course (expressed in accommodative diopter), since the focal power expressed in diopter is reversely proportional to the focal measured distance. The maximal accommodation will be the opposite of the measured distance.

The other way round works as well: "the accommodative blur technique". The reading distance is stable; we have the subject's dioptric power vary, along the same lines as the evaluation of penalization's maximum tolerated.

The text is 33 cm or 40 cm away, two possibilities:

- The subject can read the text: we add negative lenses until blur, and we note down the value of the last additional sphere diopter with which the subject could read.
- The subject cannot read the text and it is too blurred: we add positive power lenses until the subject can make the text out, and we note down the value of the additional sphere diopter enabling the reading.

It will give the maximal accommodation:

- from 33 cm by: maximal accommodation = 3.00 diopters,
- from 40 cm by: maximal accommodation = 2.50 diopters.

1.4.3.2 Duochrome Test *(Fig. 1.8)*

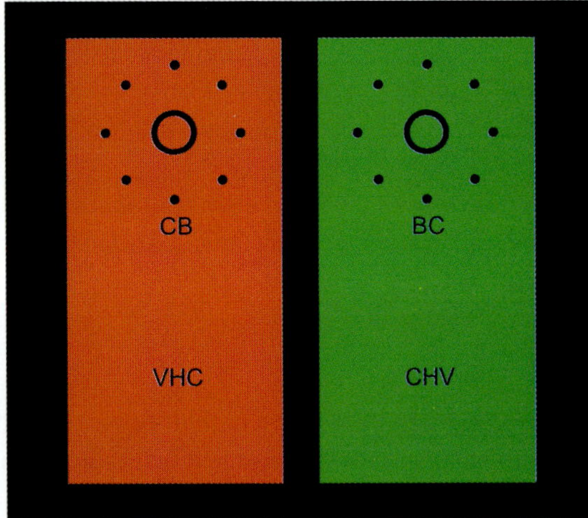

Fig. 1.8 Duochrome test (red/green) in near vision

If, without optical compensation, the reader:

- sees in the red part more clearly, it means the retina optical image of the test is focused forward,
- if he sees in the green part more clearly, it means the optical image of the test is focused at the back of the retina.

With its optical compensation, suitable for near vision, the red area should not stand out more than the green one.

The addition, thus, determined should provide the patient with clear and comfortable vision at usual reading distance.

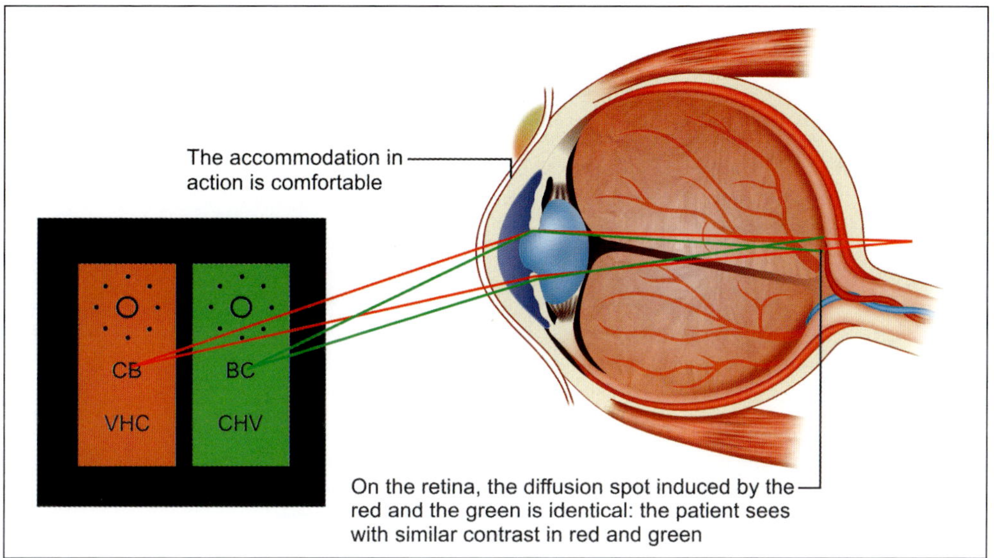

Fig. 1.9 Red-green test with equal contrast

Duochrome test lies in the optical principle of differential refraction or eye's longitudinal chromatic aberration. Chromatic differential refraction lays through a higher dioptric convergence for the shortest wavelength monochromatic lights (red) and a lower dioptric convergence for green lights (Fig. 1.9).

Consequently, a subject with balanced near-vision correction must see as clearly in the red part of the duochrome optotype, as in the green one. This test allows to screen and rebalance the optical sub or under corrections in near vision.

A typical answer about the green part translates an accommodative delay for a non-presbyope: about blacker optotypes, more contrasted, and clearer in the green. The accommodative delay for the young subject is of roughly 0.25 to 1.00 diopter.

By "accommodative delay", we mean the fact that the focus is done at the background of the test. The "young" subject is supposed to put at stake the minimal accommodation that allows him to recognize the characters that he is reading. So the smaller these characters are, the lower the accommodative delay is.

A contrary carry, an "accommodative excess" shows in a focus at the foreground of the test. The effort at stake is then inappropriate. When an accommodative excess is shown, we have to:

- determine the cause,
- know if it provokes any trouble,
- and, if needed, to solve it.

1.4.3.3 *Jackson's Cross-cylinder Test (Fig. 1.10)*

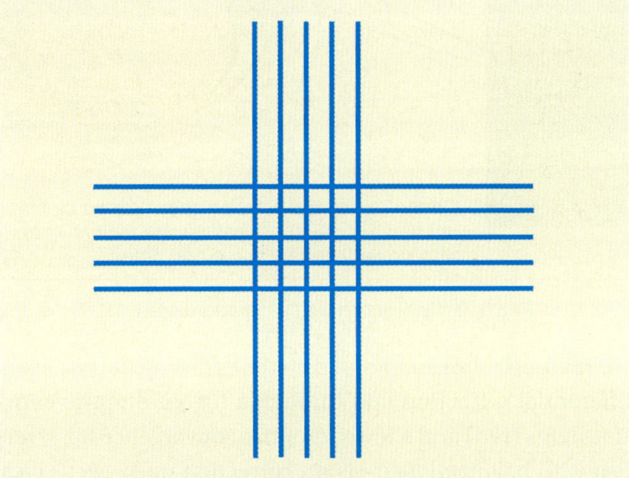

Fig. 1.10 Jackson's cross-cylinder test

Jackson's cross-cylinder is a visual test based upon the principle that, in the case of an eye with induced astigmatism, the vertical and horizontal lines are clear only at the level of the circle of least confusion. We will review this notion with the study of astigmatic presbyopia (*See also* paragraph 2.4.2, Circle of least confusion, page 64).

An accommodative delay for non-presbyope shows in an expected answer about the horizontals: said to be blacker, more contrasted, and clearer than the vertical ones. The accommodative expected delay for the young subject is of 0.25 to 1.00 diopter (Fig. 1.11).

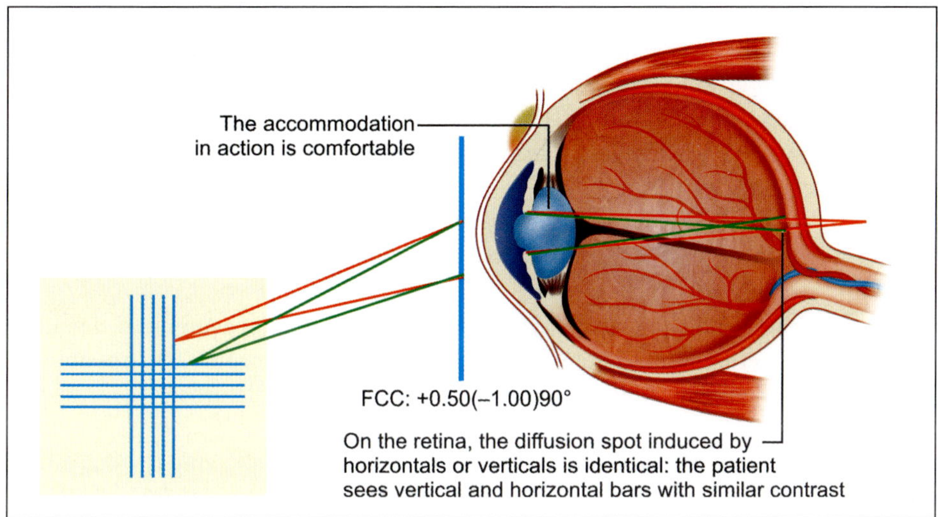

Fig. 1.11 Jackson's cross-cylinder test with equal contrast

A fixed cross-cylinder of +0.50(−1.00)90° is located forward in the ocular couple. If, without optical compensation, the reader:

- sees the verticals more clearly, it means the optical image of the test is focused forward in the retina,
- if he sees the horizontals more clearly, the test image is then focused at the back of the retina.

With its optical compensation suitable for near vision, the subject should make out the horizontals as contrasted as the verticals.

The addition thus determined is the one that will enable the patient to benefit from a clear and comfortable vision at usual reading distance.

1.4.4 Other Considerations

Is there any relationship between the far best visual acuity and the near best visual acuity? We have to know that these two visual acuities do not appeal to exactly the same anatomical structures. Indeed, if ocular discrimination power (the smallest discontinuity the eye can see) is a given subject's constant, at a given time, the patient uses different visual strategies in distance vision (scan) and in near vision (accommodation and microfluctuations so the image grows, pursuits, saccades), which prevents from establishing any equivalence between far 20/20 and near 20/20.

The optical systems can increase the size of the pictures in near vision (possibility of foveolar excentration according to the preferential loci), whereas these systems become inoperative in distance (low visions in age-related macular degeneration).

More recently, other methods of accommodation measurement have been the subject of research, especially in the United States, with the introduction of the wavefront technology; we will come back to it (*See also* paragraph 2.5.6.1, Aberrometry, page 69).

However, the only reliable and objective method of accommodation measurement, defended by Adrian Glasser, is the refractometry compared before and after instilling pilocarpine 3%, possibly instilled with phenylephrine to limit the miosis, pharmacologically induced, which disturbs measures (*See* paragraph 1.3.2, Miosis, page 13).

Normal human accommodation naturally shows microfluctuations all along the day and maybe even during sleep and certain of its phases (Rapid Eye Movement). The dominant role of the ciliary muscle during the accommodation accounts for these variations. The ciliary muscle shows electrophysiological resting potentials responsible for a kind of unceasing dynamic balance, similar to the muscular microcontractions needed for the adaptation of well-balanced postural system during static tests.

1.4.5 Accommodative Microfluctuations

It is useless to remind human eye is able to stare objects with great accuracy at different distances.

Actually, it has been proven that the eye stares slightly too close at far objects and slightly too far at the near ones.

The tension grade of the ciliary muscle, applied to increase lens refractive power when the subject fixes his gaze on a near point, varies a lot from an individual to the other.

Ciliary muscle, responsible for the accommodation, is subjected to a muscular reaction under restraint explaining microfluctuations.

The muscular charge causing fluctuations varies in accordance with the strength applied as well as the subject's vitality or state of tiredness.

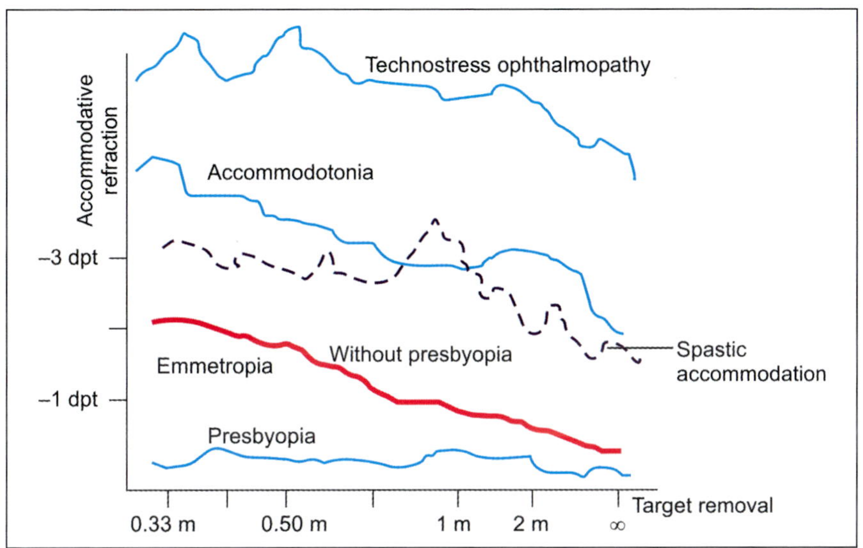

Fig. 1.12 Diagram of accommodative fluctuations in different clinical cases according to the target distance

If we analyze the tension degree of the ciliary muscle in emmetropic and non-presbyopic subject, eye refraction gradually increases as the visual targets gets closer (Fig. 1.12).

For presbyopic patients, at a distance of around 2 meters, there is some tension in the ciliary muscle but at a closer distance, it is not possible to focus anymore and the ciliary muscle does not work actively.

For the patients who have accommodotonia, focusing has an extent in accordance with the distance of the visual target; but for all distance, ciliary muscle exerts a strong tension.

In case of accommodation spasms (spastic accommodation in Figure 1.12), there is strong eye myopization and continuous tension in the ciliary muscle, without relation with the place of the visual target.

In case of technostress ophthalmopathy (Computer Vision Syndrome), the muscular tension of the ciliary muscle reacting to a distant visual target is not as important, but when the subject tries to look at a near visual target, he finds himself in pseudo-spasmodic state of accommodation.

1.5 ACCOMMODATIVE ETIOPATHOGENESIS

What are the other anatomical structures implied in accommodation, then?

To answer this delicate question, it is necessary to enter the controversial debate of accommodation mechanism and its relationships with presbyopia.

1.5.1 History

Historically speaking, and this is not always well known, it is Johannes Mueller who, in 1854 was the first to identify the ciliary body circular muscle and to theorize that its contraction produced an anterior movement of the vitreous and secondarily anterior crystalline lens displacement with increase of the refractive power.

Two years later, Herman von Helmholtz published for the first time the theory about accommodation in 74 pages in the periodical Albrecht von Graefes Arch Ophthalmol. He said the contraction of the circular ciliary muscle went together with a slackening of the tension at the level of Zinn's zonule fibers and the lens going back to its floppy rest form.

While everyone had accepted this theory, Frans Donders himself engraved it as a dogma in his 1864 work on ophthalmology.

It was not before 1924 that Lindsay Johnson recalled Helmholtz' theory into question. He argued about how unacceptable the theory was, as far as the muscular tension is concerned, since it is not usually occurring during relaxation.

As an alternative, Johnson said the change in lens curvature involved fluids compression in the circumlenticular space (*See also* paragraph 4.3.3, Ciliary exploration, page 161) during accommodation, with anterior lenticular movement and curving of the crystalline lens anterior side.

Coleman approved this theory inspired by fluids mechanism 50 years later.

The circumlenticular space is an anatomically empty space taking place: in front, by the iris posterior face, behind, by the basis of the vitreous body and the peripheral anterior vitreous cortex, outside, by ciliary processes and the zonule insertion area, and inside, by the lens equator.

Later, Coleman defended his catenary model to explain the accommodation mechanisms, by analogy with the catenary physical problem, in which a supple rope, uniformly dense and inextensible, follows the curve freely hanging by its extremities.

In 1986, he proposed to associate this curve with the anterior surface of the crystalline lens, and to liken the ciliary bodies to the pylons of a suspension bridge.

The accommodation's catenary theory refers to the catenary mathematical model:

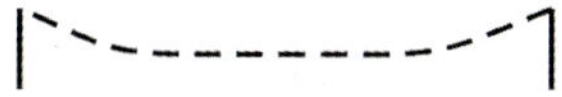

From this modelization of Coleman's catenary theory, the lenticulo-zonular complex and the anterior vitreous make up a diaphragm separating the eye anterior and posterior segments.

During the accommodation, the contraction of the ciliary muscle pushes the whole diaphragm forward in a piston moving, creating a pressure gradient between the eye two segments and leading to an anterior swelling of the crystalline lens and a flattening of its posterior face (Fig. 1.13).

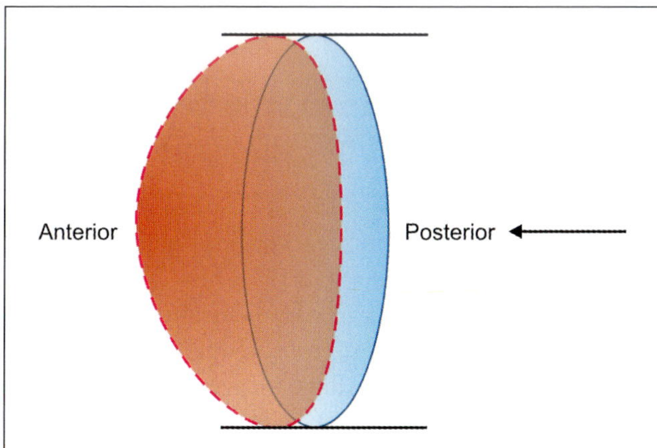

Fig. 1.13 Anterior swelling of crystalline lens and posterior flattening (leaders) in a piston movement (arrow) according to Coleman's catenary accommodation theory

1.5.2 Experimental Modelization

Experimentally, electric stimulation of a 10 volt bipolar current to a mammalian animal comes with a pressure rise of 20 cm of water (H_2O) in the anterior chamber, of 2 cm H_2O in the vitreous cavity.

This represents a pressure gradient of 5 cm H_2O between both segments, taking into account the initial pressures corrected from the differential viscosities measured in each of the compartments.

Coleman's catenary model enables to reckon on an accommodative extra from 1.80 to 2.50 diopters according to the measures of the studied eyes axial length.

The facts pleading for this catenary theory:
- the relatively non-stretch lenticular capsule,
- the presence of the vitreous to mold the crystalline lens,
- the presence of collagenous and zonular structure in the peripheral anterior vitreous, not generating equatorial forces, but tangential tractive forces at the level of crystalline lens.

The construction of a mechanical model in accordance with the catenary theory demonstrates how, during the accommodation, the crystalline lens can undergo so quick, reproducible and accurate morphological changes.

Tscherning put forward a theory diametrically opposed to Helmholtz', stipulating that the ciliary muscle contraction led to a rise in the tension of the zonular fibers then inducing a change in crystalline lens shape but not in thickness.

Back in the nineties, Schachar reopened controversy about accommodation mechanisms with an adaptation of Tscherning's theory.

In Schachar's opinion, with aging, the progressive loss of tension within the zonule would be related to a lifelong increasing equatorial lens. Having an ectodermic origin, this increase is making the zonular fibers unable to stretch the crystalline lens in its adequate shape for accommodation.

Beyond the interest of this theory, which thwarts received ideas and calls the dogmatic theories about accommodation into question, Schachar's initiative has enabled experiments, launched with modern tools to confirm or refute each hypothesis.

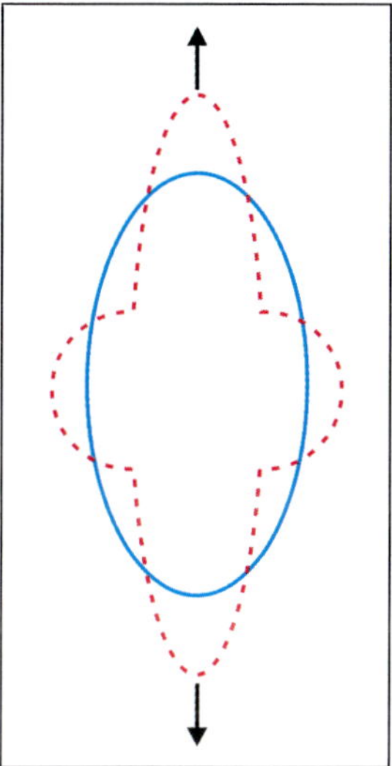

Fig. 1.14 Lenticular swelling (leaders) during accommodation (arrows) according to Schachar's theory

According to Schachar's capsular theory, the stretching of an elastic capsule comes with a mobilization of the central lenticular mass that is swelling up (Fig. 1.14).

Coleman maintains the lens capsule does not own the required biomechanical characteristics allowing the crystalline lens, not only to swell in the middle, but also to make its anterior crystalloid draw a parabolic curve while the posterior crystalloid remains unchanged.

It is then hard to believe that human beings and primates can see clearly, and within a few milliseconds, with such an elastic system.

We have underlined other breaches of the capsular theory, especially the exclusion of the vitreous role as being part of the accommodative process, and the inability to explain the translational lens moving that develops a lateral vectorial force exerted through the zonule.

Coleman cannot believe that zonule may directly exert a lateral force vector upon lens, and that ciliary muscle may show insufficient anatomical stiffness, just as the zonular bounds solidity on lenticular equator, to stretch the crystalline lens efficiently through equator.

As Thornton emphasizes it, "People believe wholeheartedly in their theory" and, like him, we reckon that all these theorists are right, somehow. Just as the accommodation would in all likelihood come from the mixture of the different mechanisms:

- increase in lenticular sphericity,
- anterior translation of crystalline lens,
- iris surrounding action,
- cerebral plasticity.

1.5.3 Clinical Approach

Moreover, we will see this further (*See also* paragraph 4.4, Accommodative experimental surgery, page 172), should the lenticular equatorial diameter increase with aging, everything that can restore the zonular tension by increasing the working distance ought to also restore accommodation (supposing that, meanwhile, the crystalline lens has not become too sclerosed).

Conversely, as some defend it, if a hardening of the crystalline lens were the main cause of presbyopia, there would be no reason for the experiments relating to the increase in circumlenticular space to be conclusive.

If these experiments were relevant, then Helmholtz would have been mistaken about the causes of presbyopia, and by extension, about the accommodation mechanism. Besides, we will see it in the therapeutic chapter (*See also* chapter 4, Presbyopia and accommodative restoration, page 136), although in an inconstant and transient manner, all the ciliary or scleral expansion surgeries have still demonstrated a subjective accommodative gain.

We have then attempted to rationalize the anatomical changes during accommodation.

Medical echographic devices use ultrasonic technology applied on the organic tissues. Ultrasounds (US) easily the soft tissues but not the aerial cavities, diffuse through which represent real obstacles for US. Melanic pigmentation or body liquids do not stop them, and their tissular penetration depends on their initial energy.

We classify the oculoechographical devices in accordance with their mode of US probes delivery:

- Mode A: propagation and linear analysis of echoes (same way as a gun bullet), which send back an image of the various met interfaces,

- Mode B: echoes bidimensional analysis (same way as a scanning), which give information about the localization of the structures on planigraphics,
- Mode C: echoes tridimensional analysis (third dimension), through spatial reconstruction of Mode B. Doppler velocimetric data that appear as colored cards for dynamic phenomena (blood flow, muscular contractility) may also enrich this mode.

Then, in a secondary step, after the anterior translation of the crystalline lens during accommodation, Mode A unidimensional echography shows a flattening of the anterior chamber, the ocular depth going from 4.09 mm in distance vision to 3.49 mm in near vision.

However, the difficulty to visualize the ciliary body and the zonular fibers, hidden behind the iris, causes many experimental biases.

Ocular albinism and aniridia clinical models, in which we can observe the entire crystalline lens by retroillumination, both contribute to Helmholtz' theory. In 1937, Fincham led studies on aniridic patients, which report a decrease of the lens equatorial diameter of about 6 to 7%, between accommodated and non-accommodated states.

We obtain magnetic resonance imaging (MRI) by the measure of the atomical magnetism developed on a body immerged in high intensity alternating magnetic field (*See also* Fig. 4.27). Each atomic nucleus that constitutes the organs (mainly Carbon, Hydrogen, Nitrogen and Oxygen) responds to this magnetic field and permits to establish anatomical slides in accordance with the observation window. Today MRI is thriving, especially in high resolution (small organs exploration) or functional imaging (imaging modifications after tests on living body).

The ocular high-resolution magnetic resonance imaging (HR MRI) allows a total visualization of the living. We can visualize:
- the iris,
- the ciliary muscle and processes,
- the crystalline lens, and
- the geometrical relationships between these different structures with no interference in iris pigmentation.

Another advantage of this technology is that it offers unequalled contrast within soft tissues, a contrast we can use to improve the observation of the tissular modifications.

With this technique, the human in vivo study on healthy volunteers aged between 22 and 91 enables, in binocular vision, to compare the accommodative performances in the physiological conditions (setting of a target at varying distance) with the pharmacologically-induced accommodation.

Some recent studies using ocular HR MRI on the rhesus monkey (Glasser) and on man (Strenk) show, unambiguously, that the crystalline lens becomes rounded during accommodation and that the equatorial diameter decreases of around 7%.

These data are incompatible with the model proposed by Schachar who states there is an increase in the equatorial diameter during the accommodation, under the effect of a greater tension that the zonule applies (*See* paragraph 1.5.2, Experimental modelization, page 30). Judging by the results of these investigations, the accommodation Helmholtz' theory thus appears to be true.

1.5.4 Accommodative Structures

The crystalline lens morphological changes, which lead to presbyopia, are less clear among the scientist community.

HR MRI leaves few doubts about the lens keeping growing with aging.

Another evidence of the continuous growth of the crystalline lens comes from the hydrated lens weight measures revealed by the human eye bank.

It is interesting to note that, at least for the human being, only the anterior part of the crystalline lens keeps growing, the equator remaining stable with aging, just as the posterior surface. However, putting the lens in the eye posterior part, this is not valid for the rhesus monkey whose lens grows in both the anterior and the posterior parts.

The growth of lens in its anterior portion results in more sphericity with aging. This leads for ciliary bodies to move forward, and then limits the possibility of a complementary anterior movement during accommodation.

A certain degree of tissular confinement (cluttering in a space anatomically closed) in the anterior segment must have an important role in presbyopia.

Although in MRI the lens equatorial diameter does not change with aging, the ciliary muscular ring obviously decreases, what lowers the zonular tension down to zero in non-accommodated state.

Given its position in the annular part, ciliary muscle acts as a real muscular diaphragm, the contraction of which provokes a decrease of the eye transversal diameter.

The ciliary muscular ring moving inward under the effect of the zonule seems more plausible.

Nevertheless, MRI claims that this ciliary displacement does not come with any amyotrophy since the contractile activity persists whatever the age.

As the lens grows, the axial thickness increasing, the zonular fibers seem to slacken, without the crystalline lens becoming loose or unstable with aging.

Effectively, an unstable lens would imply accommodation microfluctuations for the older, which is not the case.

The data given by MRI show the uveal tract solidarily reacts as an answer to the growing lenticular thickness in presbyopia.

While we admit the lens hardness increases with aging, the data of a study led by Weeber show there is an exponential increase of the lenticular resistivity with aging that could accompany the accommodation linear decrease.

The Dutch researcher Weeber settles the basis of a nonuniform lens biophysical model, integrating a finished succession of anatomical elements that define a gradient of resistivity.

This model comes from the data of dynamic mechanical analysis made to measure the lens total resistivity, as well as its segmentary resistivity, on subjects recently deceased and aged between 18 and 90.

The results show a change in lens global resistivity and inside, the appearance of a gradient of resistivity with aging.

While putting that crystalline lens is a homogeneous structure and only by keeping the global resistivity, accommodation should linearly decrease with aging at around 1 diopter per decade.

However, if we modelize the lens as a heterogeneous structure with the appearance of a resistivity gradient with aging, we obtain an accommodation change curve according to the age in the shape of a sigmoid (Fig. 1.15).

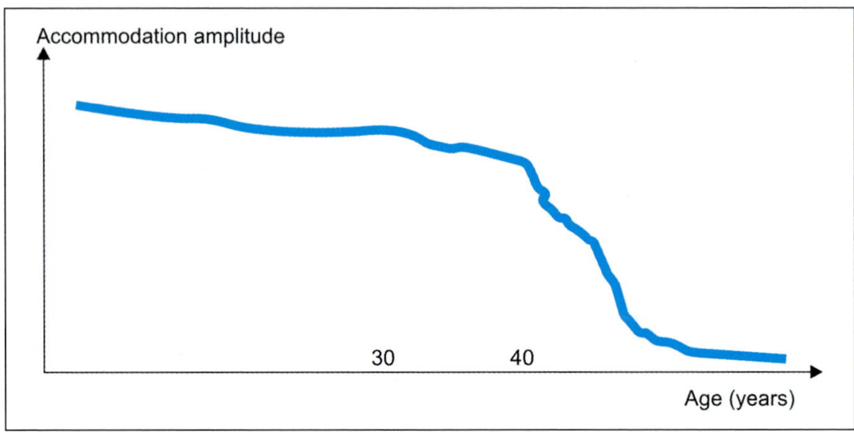

Fig. 1.15 Accommodation change curve according to age

Firstly, this curve shows an initial slow decline of the accommodation amplitude between 30 and 40, secondly, a quicker drop during the next decade, and finally, a progressive decline between 50 and 60, until reaching another steady state.

We can use this new discovery about lens differential resistivity changes to explain why the aging crystalline lens loses its capacity to change its shape during accommodation.

The resistivity differentials can also permit to modelize a referential frame of the accommodative amplitude changes according to the age, as close as possible to clinical data that we have noted during the progressive settlement of presbyopia.

The dynamic mechanical analysis of lens resistivity measurement has the advantage of providing information about the lens viscoelastical properties.

In order to determine the segmentary resistivity, the investigators have cut the lenses along the equatorial plane and have proceeded with localized microprobes. The measures they obtain have integrated the mathematical Shear Modulus (modulus of rigidity) and Young's Modulus (modulus of elasticity), then enabling to show the exponential increase of the resistivity with aging.

The results of the segmentary resistivities study point that both the nucleus and the cortex become more resistant with aging.

Nonetheless, the magnitude of change differs for these two structures and is clearly greater for the nucleus than for the cortex.

In all the samples of crystalline lens measured, the nuclear resistivity grows by a factor of 10,000 where cortical resistivity only increases by 100.

The crystalline lens nucleus seems tenfold softer than the cortex in a young lens, with a resistivity relatively uniform around 50 years old, while the nucleus has a resistivity 200 times greater at the level of the cortex in older samples.

The mechanical model of finite elements used to describe the accommodation amplitude takes into account:

- the crystalline lens,
- the capsular bag and
- a part of the zonular apparatus.

On different studies of the human myopia pathogenesis, some authors studied the ocular biometrical changes during the accommodation.

The ocular axial length increases by 60 μm with 3 diopters of accommodation, and by around 120 μm for 8 diopters.

An eyeball axial extension of 12.7 μm added with 5.1 accommodation diopters tallies with a change of the total power of the eye of –0.036 diopters.

The contraction of the ciliary muscle, linked with an anterior and internal movement of choroid and sclera, may induce ocular elongation, occurring during accommodation.

1.5.5 Pseudo-accommodation

After this presentation of the actual debate about accommodation and the origin of presbyopia, it is essential to distinguish accommodation from pseudo-accommodation.

Effectively, understanding the difference between these two entities is paramount to deal with ametropic presbyopia, as well as assessing the success of therapeutic approaches of presbyopia.

Remind that the components of the proper accommodation are:
- the axial lens movement (Mueller),
- the increase of the sphericity (Helmholtz),
- the lens swelling (Schachar),
- the piston effect (Coleman),
- the convergence-miosis synkinesis, and
- the dynamic extension of the ocular axial length.

To quote only the elements we have already studied [see previous paragraphs].

If we take them separately, each of these elements produce a partial accommodation, but not a pseudo-accommodation.

Pseudo-accommodation is connected with astigmatism (*See also* paragraph 2.4, Presbyopia and astigmatisms, page 60), for instance, or the pinhole effect (*See* paragraph 1.3.2, Miosis, page 13), or a corneal multifocality (*See also* paragraph 3.3.7, PresbyLASIK, page 103), produced intentionally or not.

Optically speaking we usually consider cornea as neutral during accommodation.

Nevertheless, some authors, by the observation of a corneal accommodation in chicken, have called into question the role of the cornea during accommodation.

Since cornea has a major refractive role in the eye (*See* paragraph 1.2.2, Various enlarger systems in vertebrates, page 4), subtle changes in the power of the cornea center during the accommodation can be sufficient to play a part in modifying the ocular total optical power.

If we could demonstrate that the cornea played a part in the accommodative process, we should thus exclude this anatomical element from the pseudo-accommodation field.

According to Yasuda, there are many modifications of the corneal curvature, which videokeratotopography confirmed, during accommodation.

Is this about a passive training of the sclerocorneal limbus (anatomically linked with the ciliary muscle via the scleral spur and the trabecular filter)? (*See also* Fig. 4.25).

Is it about an indirect effect linked with the pressural modifications or with a cyclotorsion effect during accommodation?

The corneal curvature increases with the ciliary muscle contraction, with, therefore, an increase of the refractive power between 0.60 and 0.72 diopter during accommodation.

A light corneal accommodative effect seems to be bound with the anatomical close relationship between the corneal periphery and ciliary muscle.

The instilling of high-dose pilocarpine (4%) to induce accommodation pharmacologically comes with topographic curvature change, with no cyclotorsion, in the first 30 minutes while we have not even measured the pressural effect.

1.5.6 Compared Imaging of Accommodation

The compared physiology with modern imaging techniques permitted to better apprehend the accommodative phenomena peculiar to humans.

Because of the iris hampering all direct observation of the ciliary muscle in intact human's eye, many attempts to study the ciliary muscle accommodative behavior are based on in vivo and in vitro animal's data (especially in rhesus monkey) and upon in vitro human studies.

In primates (monkeys, humans) accommodative systems, happen to be similar on many points, but very dissimilar as for the accommodative loss with aging.

Inter-species differences do exist in crystalline lens development and its physiological growth, which leads to significant differences in geometrical interconnections between:

- the ciliary muscle and
- the crystalline lens and the corresponding vectorial forces implied in the accommodative mechanisms.

Even in the aging of the ciliary muscle remain inter species differences, from what the probable differences of development of presbyopia in rhesus monkey and human.

For example, the human ciliary muscle contraction does not decrease with aging (*See* paragraph 1.5.4, Accommodative structures, page 34), as opposed to the monkey's ciliary muscle that shows a reduction of the contractile answer with aging, certainly due to choroidal modifications (this contraction restores after it frees from its posterior choroid ties).

Moreover, while the human ciliary muscle apex makes an anterior displacement with aging, the rhesus' ciliary muscle remains at an obvious posterior location in the eye.

With accommodation, monkey's ciliary muscle simultaneously makes anterior and inward displacements, whereas the human's one only moves inward during accommodation.

Finally, the studies in microscopy indicate the aging human ciliary muscle develops more connective tissue—and in more muscle anatomical areas—than the monkey.

With the wealth of these inter-species differences, the strategies of presbyopic correction working for monkey can then turn ineffective for man.

The fact that the human ciliary muscle contraction does not decrease with aging, remains true for the phakic or posterior chamber pseudophakic subject, at advanced stage of presbyopia.

Though the presbyope's ciliary muscle contracts as much as in young, we notice a significant decrease of the ciliary muscular ring diameter in phakic or pseudophakic presbyope.

Because the lens equatorial diameter, on a non-accommodated eye, is stable with aging, a proportional decrease of the ciliary muscular ring diameter with aging leads to a shrinking of circumlenticular space (*See* paragraph 1.5.1, History, page 28) and a drop in zonular tension in non-accommodated phakic eye.

To the most advanced stage of presbyopia, the zonular tension can reach zero in non-accommodated state, what shows through a muscular ciliary contraction unable to diminishing a ciliary tension already nil.

These choroidal aspects help explain how presbyopia appears in monkey, but this has not been enough for human since the accommodative ciliary muscular contraction is set for life.

As we will see this (*See also* paragraph 3.3.9, Lenticular surgeries, page 109), it goes the same for the movements observed in the pseudophakic implanted patients with so-called accommodative artificial crystalline lenses where the ciliary muscle and choroid-dependent strengths are efficient, even in advanced presbyopia.

1.5.7　Lens Equator Growth and Accommodative Amplitude

Between 18 and 50 years old, the accommodation amplitude invariably decreases at a near linear speed of 0.3 diopters a year.

However, during childhood, the accommodative amplitude decreases much quicker between 5 and 10 years old, at a speed twice greater than in teenagers.

This fast decline in accommodation amplitude during childhood is a track to understand the fall of accommodative amplitude with aging.

We cannot explain the rapid drop of accommodation amplitude during childhood by a structural modification of:

- the cornea,
- the axial length, even if the measures by OCT show a change of up to 12 µm during accommodation,
- the ciliary musculature and the zonule, and
- the neurosensory innervation.

On the other hand, the quick fall in accommodative amplitude during childhood could become clearer if we take into account the great changes in geometrical properties and content of crystalline lens.

We generally propose that a modification in hardness and resistivity of the lens nucleus might be responsible for presbyopia. Nonetheless, neither lens hardness nor resistivity undergoes any change during childhood (*See* paragraph 1.5.4, Accommodative structures, page 34).

Actually, with the use of approved parallel-plate rheometer to measure the accurate viscoelastical figures, we demonstrated that the hardness and/or resistivity of fresh human lens nuclei, obtained from volunteer and deceased donors aged less than 40, were not correlated with aging.

Moreover, the clinical observation corroborated these experimental data, as long as the lens optical density (*See also* Fig. 3.5) remained unchanged until 40 years old and the lens natural yellowing is not correlated with the accommodative amplitude.

Nevertheless, the lens capsule regularly thickens and hardens during the three first decades in life, whereas it modifies very little during childhood.

We describe a coating tissue to the crystalline lens called lenticular capsule:

- anterior capsule,
- posterior capsule.

The increase in capsular hardness and resistivity happens to increase indeed the efficiency of the zonular tension, which does not constitute any element to explain the drop in accommodative amplitude.

If we now pay attention to the lens central thickness, it decreases during the first two decades of life and slowly increases shortly thereafter: in fact, regarding this biphasic evolution, the lenticular nucleus responsibility for the decline in accommodative amplitude with aging is unlikely.

As all the ectodermal tissues do, the whole lenticular stroma grows all along its life.

The lenticular stroma is made of lens fibers that developed from epithelial cells located in lens equatorial region; as a result the equatorial lenticular diameter increases with aging *(See* paragraph 1.5.2, Experimental modelization, page 30).

The lens equatorial diameter grows following a logarithmic model (Fig. 1.16):
- quickly during the first two decades of life,
- and then slowly after 30.

Zonule connects the lens equator with the ciliary muscle. There is no argument for a modification with aging. Therefore, as the lens equatorial diameter increases with aging, there is a decrease with aging in the basic length of ciliary muscle.

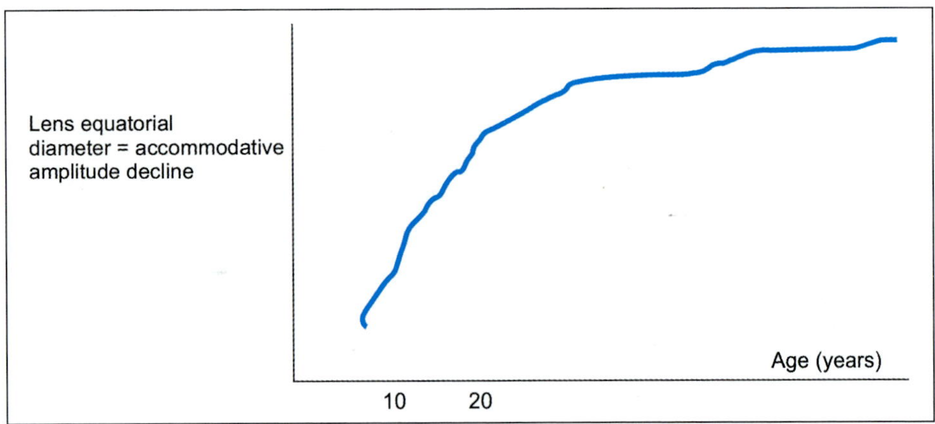

Fig. 1.16 Increase in lens equatorial diameter and in decline of accommodative amplitude depending on age

Since all the muscles follow a rule between length and tension, and as the basic length decreases, the maximum amount of force the ciliary muscle displays tends to go down and cause an accommodative amplitude loss with aging.

Since the lens equatorial diameter increases rapidly during childhood, the basic length decreases quickly at that time, this period being responsible for the fast decline in accommodation all childhood long.

After the two first decades of life, the lens equatorial diameter increases slowly, so much that, between 18 and 50 years old, the basic length of the ciliary muscle decreases linearly, just as the decline in accommodation amplitude.

1.5.8 Decrease of Accommodative Amplitude on Intraocular Pressure (IOP)

Equatorial lenticular growth follows a logarithmic curve (*See* paragraph 1.5.7, Lens equator growth and accommodative amplitude, page 40) that also forecast the growth profile of intraocular pressure (IOP) with aging.

Scleral spur (*See also* Fig. 4.25) links ciliary muscle and trabecular network together. An increase in the ciliary muscular tonus extends the flow of aqueous humor leading to a fall in IOP.

Thereby, the lens equatorial growth brings about changes in the basic length of the muscle ciliary that are likely to affect the basic IOP.

For the lens equatorial diameter increases in accordance with a logarithmic progress, IOP should also increase logarithmically.

Indeed, IOP logarithmically increases with aging, rapidly during childhood, then slowly.

Actually, the outcome of IOP exactly matches the logarithmic increase of the lens equatorial growth.

Normally, the lens equatorial growth guides the decline with aging of the accommodative amplitude that clinically appears in presbyopia from the fifth decade of life and comes with an increase in IOP as well.

Besides, with the strength of those considerations that permit to better understand the actual relationships between accommodation and presbyopia, it is about time to leave emmetropic accommodative physiology for the place of presbyopia in various ocular pathologies disorders and in refractive (spherocylindrical ametropias) (*See also* chapter 2, Presbyopia and ametropias, page 44).

Presbyopia and Ametropias

As we saw this previously (*See also* paragraph 1.2.3, Accommodative involution, page 9), presbyopia affects all the people aged 38 to 40 and older.

We estimate that on an international basis, the subjects without refractive problem (emmetropes) are dispatched only one out of four, the three remaining quarters being as follows:

- 2 hyperopias/4 people (included with an astigmatism),
- 1 myopia/4 people (included with astigmatism).

However odd these proportions may seem, and from a finalist viewpoint, nature has followed the rule commonly called "distant vision normality", but has favored hyperopic ametropia, the vision we find the most in predators (*See also* paragraph 1.2.1, Compared ontogeny, page 4).

An ametropia is a refractive dysfunction, generally non-pathological one. The optical image of a far object, when the accommodation is relaxed, does not appear on the retina (*See also* Fig. 1.7). We distinguish the spherical ametropias from the astigmatisms (cylindrical or non-spherical ametropias).

In a population coming from our eye centers, the study of presbyopia must then takes these statistics into account. Indeed, at the age of presbyopia, hyperopes and myopes face completely different problems.

Nonetheless, we have to admit that if the refraction vices represent the cornerstone of our speciality, numerous ophthalmologists, opticians, orthoptists, optometrists are unaware of the existing relationship between these ametropias and presbyopia. Besides, it is even harder to get a good idea of this connection since there is no progress table, no reference system.

For the most, we can depict some important points about the natural tendencies of each ametropia to evolve and integrate presbyopia, with more or less difficulties. This is the purpose of this very chapter.

On different stages, all these refraction troubles can come with some ophthalmological or general pathologies that can also influence presbyopia starting, development and treatment.

Let us mention this chapter excludes all other affection altering the integrity of the visual envelope, even though these can have impact on presbyopia. For example, we would not come to visual field abnormalities, color sense abnormalities, vision abnormalities related to light intensity, perception errors, or visual agnosia.

All the ophthalmological pathology likewise can have a knock-on effect on presbyopia whether at the level of:

- eyebrows (inflammatory lesion),
- eyelashes (hypertrichosis),
- eyelids (position abnormalities),
- palpebral aperture (ptosis),
- lacrimal apparatus (lacrimation),
- orbit (dystopia),
- eyeball (phthisis bulbi),
- ocular tonus (glaucoma),
- caruncle or plica semilunaris (tumor),
- sclerotic episcleral conjunctiva (pterygion),
- cornea (opacities),
- anterior chamber (hyphema),
- iris (atrophy),
- pupil (mydriasis),
- crystalline lens (cataract),
- vitreous (hyalitis),
- ocular fundus (maculopathy),
- uvea (uveitis),
- oculo-palpebral sensitivity (hypoesthesia),
- palpebral motility (blepharospasm), ocular motility (palsies),
- visual axis disjunction (spasms),
- gaze fixing abnormalities (tics),
- head malpositions caused by the eye (torticollis).

Naturally, we will only evoke these pathologies when they have an immediate connection with presbyopia, for it is not about carrying out comprehensive testbook of ophthalmology.

2.1 PRESBYOPIA AND EMMETROPIA (Fig. 2.1)

The refraction vice is defined as a fall in distant visual acuity, when accommodation is nil, able to improve with optical compensation (spectacles, lenses, surgery).

The absence of refraction error—etymologically emmetropia (emmetropia)—defines as a clear far vision without accommodative effort.

This is why the notions of the previous chapter obviously are to study the refraction troubles (*See also* chapter 1, Accommodation and presbyopia, page 1).

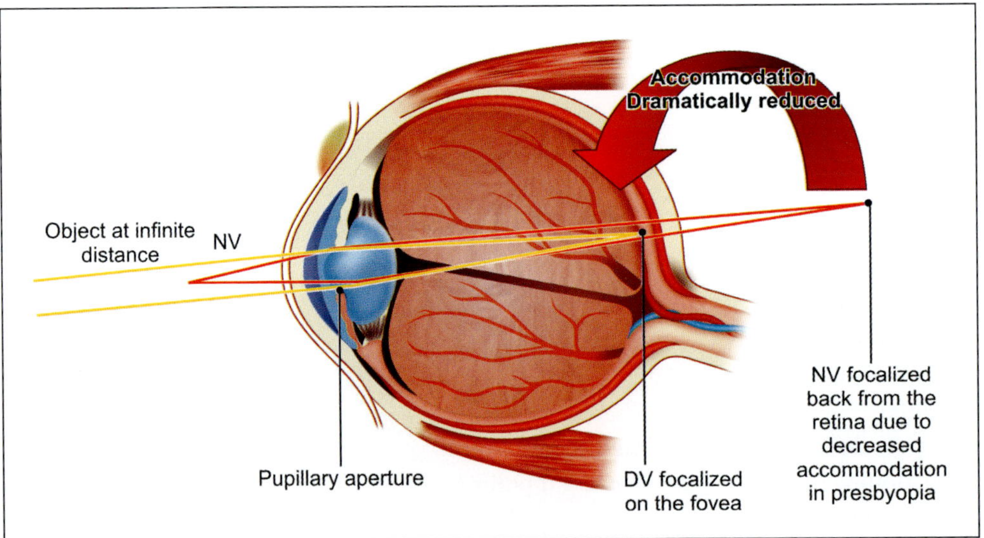

Fig. 2.1 Presbyopia in emmetropes' distant vision (DV), near vision and accommodation in not compensated near vision

In not compensated presbyopic emmetropia, the accommodation amplitude in near vision (NV), does not allow the subject to see clearly anymore. This being due to the focal image which does not appear on the foveal plan, but at the back of it.

Effectively, emmetropes focus the image on their fovea in distant vision, without any accommodative effort, what does not exclude possible accommodative fluctuations between balance position (microfluctuations) (*See also* paragraph 1.4.5, Accommodative microfluctuations, page 26) with hazards of life (fatigue, personal and professional stress, anxiety).

Those fluctuations, which our young patients consider very annoying in their daily life, tend to decrease as they age until completely disappearing after about 50 years old.

2.2 PRESBYOPIA AND HYPEROPIA

Let us then consider the case of hyperopias (most frequently ametropia in statistics) and see how presbyopia changes both hyperopes vision and life.

Hypermetropia (or hyperopia) is a static refraction abnormality from which the image of a point located to infinity appears at the back of the retina.

2.2.1 Hyperopic Compensation

This explains the progressive decompensation of hyperopia and the need for an optical compensation first in NV, and then in DV at the age of presbyopia (Fig. 2.2).

This last point is crucial for hyperopes, for it defines what we call the natural compensation. When a hyperope naturally compensates his trouble, he does not show any sign.

The visual fall is inconstant and this point is of utmost importance for it conditions the trouble unawareness among our patients. It is difficult to have hyperopes admit a correction, while they have a handicap they do not even feel, or very slightly. This explains the time it takes to the hyperopic subject to accept a compensation for he does so only when he largely decompensates his trouble.

The visual fall is variable for hyperopes. It regards both near and distant vision, or near only, according to the possibilities of compensation by means of accommodation.

We have to distinguish in congenital constitutional hyperopias:
* the form known as primitive, axile-type simple hyperopia, most of the time hereditary with predominant autosomal transmission (moderate hyperopias), or autosomal recessive (high hyperopias) and,

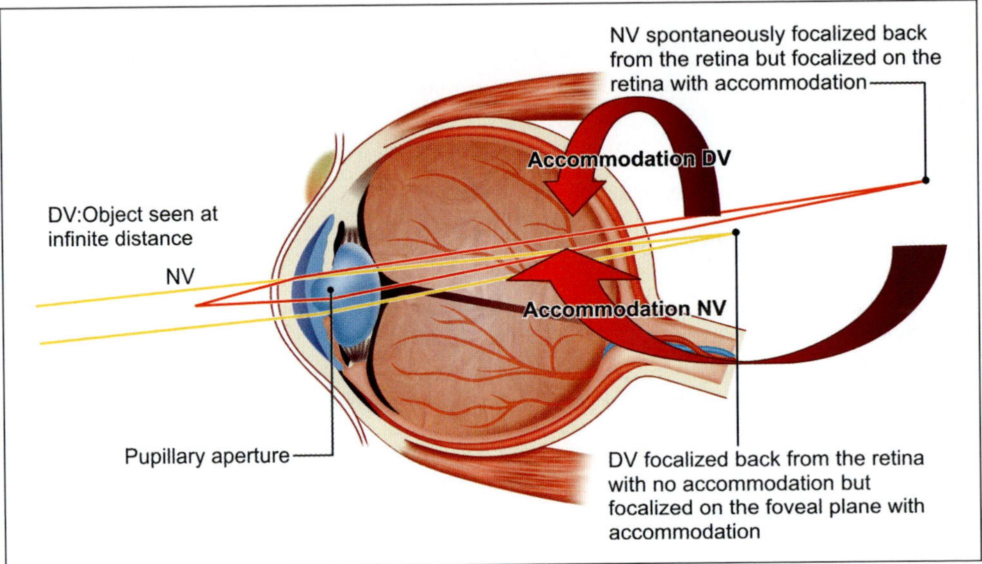

Fig. 2.2 Distant vision, near vision and accommodation in optically not compensated hyperopic patient

In no corrected hyperopes, the distant-vision (DV) accommodation is necessary to maintain a clear image on the retina. Near vision (NV) needs an even greater accommodation amplitude.

- the secondary form or linked with various ocular malformations (microphthalmia, cornea plana, microcornea, ectopia lentis, lens coloboma) often hypoplasia or macula-associated aplasia. Hyperopia is usually bilateral and more or less symmetrical, except for acquired hyperopias.

The unilateral, axile, acquired hyperopia may be secondary to local causes or orbital affections like:
- orbital tumors lying in retrobulbar cone,
- intraocular tumors interesting anterior pole,
- idiopathic retinal detachments or chorioretinal or secondary retinal detachments, leaking in macular region,
- some retinal detachment surgeries (with reduction of the scleral surface),
- ocular hypotonia.

Some scars, corneal flattening, whether traumatically-induced or not (sequelae of superficial or deep keratitis) can be responsible for curvature hyperopia:

- posterior dislocations or in the crystalline lens frontal plane,
- aphakia and lens dislocation,
- certain cortical cataracts,
- some iridocyclitis are responsible for an index hyperopia,
- just as some general causes like diabetes (hyperopia coming with a peak of hyperglycemia), or hydrocarbon diet.

As we will see it, there is a study of the simple or compound hyperopic astigmatisms (*See* Fig. 2.5); we will then stand in the general case of pure primitive hyperopias, without astigmatism.

In physiological optics, it is due to the relatively too short hyperopic eye, compared with the ocular diopters, that the focal image is located at the back of the foveal plane. This explains the need to use optical systems to compensate converging dioptrical values (positive), in order to bring the focal image back in the foveal plane.

As a matter of fact, the dioptrical value necessary for this compensation to be efficient depends on the extent of the underlying hyperopia.

2.2.2 Pediatric Hyperopia

Let us emphasize again the need to free young hyperopes from accommodation (frequent instilling of cycloplegic, as we have studied it in the previous chapter (*See* paragraph 2.2.1, Hyperopic compensation, page 47), in young hyperopes) to objectively assess the hyperopic value.

Effectively, if we remember that accommodation decreases with aging, it is imperative to examine babies and children with tropicamide (speed and short time action), cyclopentolate (active within 45 minutes to an hour but prolonged for several hours) or with atropine or its derivatives (effect after 1 or 2 hours but persisting for quite a long time, up to several days).

Conversely, an ophthalmopediatric examination without instillation of cycloplegics may be very uncertain to conclude about refraction, all the more since the patient is young and hardly hyperopic.

The notion of high, moderate or low hyperopia takes into account:

- not only the thickness of the ophthalmic lenses, which the patient always wears too thick, hence the making of ultra-thin lenses, but also,

- the visual handicap the patient feels, or even,
- the frequency of the associated pathologies (acute glaucoma).

In practice, low hyperopias are +2.00 diopters inferior to an aerial correction (spectacles lenses), moderate hyperopias are between an aerial correction of +2.00 and +4.00 diopters, high hyperopias are beyond +4.00 diopters.

From birth onwards, the small size of the ocular globe frequently makes a moderate hyperope of the infant, however his extraordinary accommodative power (up to 20 diopters, as we saw it in the previous chapter) (*See also* paragraph 1.4.3.1, Search for maximal accommodation, page 21), allows him to maintain a hyperopia measured between +1.00 and +3.00 diopters.

Taking into account the frequent genetical transmission of this refraction default, we advise the parents who have the affection to refer their children, however asymptomatic they may be, for a baby vision test between 8 and 9 months old (infant screening test).

Too often, ophthalmologists examine babies aged 11 months or more, which is a rather challenging age for a relevant exam prior to verbalization (around 3 years old).

Because, let us remind it, unilateral amblyopia (an eye with weaker acuity than the other, the ocular couple being perfectly compensated) might develop only, in children who reach 6 and a half years old, because of health carelessness. At this age, amblyopia becomes irreversible, what was still relatively reversible before 6, thanks to optical correction and an appropriate treatment.

In human, this "sensitive period" of vision development stretches until around 8 to 10 years of age, but its border line remains unclearly defined. Moreover, the risk for an amblyopia to appear is all the more important since the child is younger (between 1 and 4 years old).

This affection can be reversible if we propose an appropriate re-education early enough. That re-education is even more so effective since we do it earlier, but becomes almost impossible or very hard after 7. Extract from the French book "*La malvoyance chez l'adulte: la comprendre, la vivre mieux*", Vuibert éditions, France.

For visual screening, refer bright infants around 7 to 8 months, and calm babies when they are around 9 to 10 months.

Baby screening test is based upon the preferential gazing technique. Test occurs with a child, one eye hidden, in arms of his parent, and the examiner behind a "Punch-and-Judy-Show" theater, showing him acuity cards that are more and more selective.

Although rough, this exam enables to define a normal acuity for the considered age, and above all to check the isoacuity between both eyes (quest of amblyopias). This exam comes together with an extensive ophthalmological research.

With growing, child axial hyperopia decreases as well as its accommodative power, so much that the "normal" young child remains hyperopic until he is 6, and tends towards emmetropia from his tenth year.

In clinical practice, low hyperopia during puberty has slight chances to disappear afterwards.

If, for reasons of accommodative compensation, the pubescent child spontaneously gives up his optical correction, it is to certainly to get it back with the symptoms of ocular tiredness he might feel again (between 20 and 30).

2.2.3 High Hyperopia

As for high hyperopia, accommodation only can not compensate it, with no patent functional sign (accommodative strabismus) since its value often exceeds +4.00 diopters.

Ever since he was a child, a high hyperope has been aware of his distant and near vision handicap that he can feel all the time since, contrary to a myope (we will see it later) (*See* paragraph 2.3.1, Myopias, page 55), he can not do without an optical compensation.

The peculiar case of aphakia (lack of crystalline lens owning itself a converging optical power from +18.00 to +20.00 diopters) is quite caricatural. Aphakia indeed leads the subject to abruptally suffer from a high hyperopia and dramatic presbyopia.

Judging by the patient's initial ametropia, a myopia of –5.00 diopters will lead to an expected +15.00 refraction in the aphake, an initial hyperopia of +2.00 will lead to a refraction of +22.00 in the aphake, meaning the corrective lens is of significant thickness.

As we will see it later (*See* paragraph 2.2.4, Optical compensation, page 52), this gives rise to specific optical problems to consider a correction of presbyopia in aphakia.

With a wealth of this refractive experience, moderate hyperopes and emmetropes are the happiest until the starting point of presbyopia.

Hyperopic refractive examination, above all before the 3rd decade, must free from accommodation to only compensate the hyperopic trouble. For this doing, the technique of the blur method is essential. It can avoid the instilling of cycloplegic drops, which are very disabling.

The technique of examining via refractive blur is about systematically overcompensating the examined subject. Adding more than 1 diopter so as to limit the natural accommodation, then being inoperative and minimized.

We start the reading test with the biggest letters, what gives the hyperopes enough time to let their accommodation rest.

We then try to maintain this accommodative rest until the end of the exam, while progressively reducing of a quarter the value of the lenses before the eye each time the letters are too blurred.

The best way to make the exam is behind an automated refractor making the restriction of the latency period possible in between the different lens powers we use.

It is important to notice that, with the coming of automatic autorefractometers in our offices, subjective refraction in hyperopes is often underestimated because of a natural accommodation behind the optics of measurement.

It is all but scarce to find a negative dioptric value in the case of a low hyperopia as automatic refraction.

We thus have to carry out the blurring method in monocular and in binocular and not to hesitate to start the test with high value positive lenses.

2.2.4 Optical Compensation

Most often, hyperopia is evolving until puberty, before a period of stability during which we can propose different treatments, we will come back to this (*See also* paragraph 3.3, Presbyopia and refractive surgeries, page 93).

Accommodation at stake for these subjects to obtain a clear vision in all distance is often superior to the available comfortable accommodation.

This may cause an "exhaustion effect". From 37 to 38 years old (sometimes earlier, according to the value of the hyperopia), after overwork, presbyopic hyperopes may feel increasing tiredness all along the day, or the week, but which is reversible, during vacation or resting times.

These low hyperopes do not stand having to wear an optical compensation in intermediate vision (computer screen) and near vision (read, write), but, constrained, they do submit themselves. Although at first, they still generally refuse all compensation in far vision:

"In the distance, I do not need any optical correction" is what they often tell me in consultation.

Actually, the decrease reading performance in dark conditions confirms the handicap condition induced by ametropia: decreasing more or less visible in their distant visual acuity.

This is why it may be judicious, during summer to encourage them to wear glasses progressively—and why not tinted ones–. We will see it in the chapter about treatments (*See also* paragraph 3.1.2, Customized spectacles, page 82).

Hyperopes often ask whether they should rather free themselves from all near vision correction in order to delay the evolution of presbyopia. As ophthalmologists, we have to advise widely the wearing of spectacles in near vision, as soon as the slightest fatigue or trouble is felt.

If we consider hyperopic accommodative potential, and so that we avoid all dogmatic prescription, we will advise only hyperopes with high accommodative reserve to wear ophthalmic lenses occasionally. As opposed to the subjects with lower accommodative reserve that should do so more frequently.

Likewise we can optimize the environment:

- inciting patients to adjust the intensity and the quality of the surrounding lights in order to help the natural compensation of the subject,
- avoiding colored or insufficiently contrasted inscriptions and pages,
- minimizing the use of glazed paper,
- then favoring a good screen contrast, appropriate font and satisfactory ergonomy of the work station (monitor lower than horizontal from the eyes viewpoint, indirect light, natural light coming from the side).

In doing so, we indeed put the incidence of the evolution of presbyopia back a few months, even if, afterwards, the fall in near vision happens to be more brutal.

At this stage of early presbyopia, hyperopes claim a deterioration of their visual trouble, most often by steps.

Nevertheless, we sometimes confirm a slow and regular worsening, which compels us to change the optical correction more frequently.

It is then very important to prescribe the most saturated near minimal addition in distant vision, in hyperopes (meaning having the convex maximum); we will come back to this (*See also* paragraph 3.1.1, Addition determining, page 80).

Compensating ametropia with the convex maximum (or concave minimum) comes down to prescribing the most positive compensation, which gives the best acuity, in binocular vision.
- For hyperopes, this is "the most positive" equipment.
- For myopes, this is "the least negative" one.

Along with the inescapable evolution of his presbyopia, hyperopes will see their optical compensation value change every 2 to 4 years, to reach a stable top around 63 years old.

We will notice that, in time and with accommodation decrease, in time, hyperopes better tolerates optical correction saturated in distant vision. This comes with a slight progression of the optical compensation of presbyopia.

We have to give up on monofocality in time to advise multifocal apparatus, as soon as the hyperopic subject asks for it as he needs it in his professional or leisure activities.

There is a frequent confusion that hyperopes themselves make, as for the component of presbyopia and hyperopia in their visual trouble.

Here is what the conflictual relationship between hyperopia and the emergence of presbyopia are like in the hyperopic natural history.

It is completely different for the myopic subjects who feel the constraints coming together with presbyopia less rapidly than hyperopes.

2.3 PRESBYOPIA AND MYOPIA

Myopia is a spherical ametropia that shows through a decrease in distant visual acuity more or less significant, whereas the near or very near visual acuity persists under cycloplegia (*See also* paragraph 1.3.4, Accommodative insufficiencies, page 15).

We distinguish:
- axial myopia,
- curvature myopia,
- index myopia.

Congenital and primitive forms are generally the axial type. Congenital myopia is sometimes due to:
- a prematurity ("pepper-and-salt" aspect or retina paleness, possible retinopathy),
- a fetopathy (syphilis, congenital toxoplasmosis, pregnancy-induced toxemia, irradiation), or genetically-induced.

2.3.1 Myopias

Primitive myopia generally appears during childhood, or teenagers.

It is hereditary, with predominant autosomal transmission. Moderate myopias come with recessive autosomal transmission and high myopias with mostly recessive autosomal transmission.

High myopias show associate signs such as:
- low accommodative amplitude,
- convergence insufficiency or excess.

They can also be related to the presence of:
- open angle glaucoma,
- choroidal cataract,
- myopic choroidosis (mostly observed in high myopias),
- single conus (mostly temporal) or double one (in peripapillary ring),
- peripheral degenerative alterations (mainly temporal ones) of variable type (white or cystoid lattice degeneration),
- macular hemorrhage sometimes with pigment secondary Fuchs' stain,
- pericentral (and often central) tracks of chorioretinal atrophy that spread more or less widely, of variable shape, often with pigment proliferation,
- hemorrhages,
- breaks of Bruch's membrane, sometimes secondary idiopathic retinal detachment.

We can also connect myopia with:
- essential nyctalopia,
- Fuchs atrophia gyrata,
- chorioretinal heredodegenerations,
- central choroid sclerosis,

- Wagner's syndrome of hyaloidoretinal degeneration,
- nystagmus and amblyopia,
- congenital external ophthalmoplegia,
- generalized or ocular albinism,
- congenital spondyloepiphyseal dysplasia,
- cerebro-ocular dysplasia (Krause's syndrome),
- Cervenka's syndrome,
- homocystinuria,
- Minkowski-Chauffard disease,
- Sorsby's congenital poikiloderma,
- Amalric's syndrome,
- Aberfeld's syndrome,
- Kartagener's syndrome,
- Cornelia de Lange's syndrome,
- Apert's syndrome,
- status dysraphicus,
- Alport's syndrome,
- arachnodactylia,
- congenital anhidrotic ectodermal dysplasia,
- Rubinstein-Taybi syndrome,
- Bourneville's tuberous sclerosis,
- Norman-Landing disease,
- syndromes with chromosomal aberration (XXXX, XXYY, XXXXY, complex mosaic of sexual chromosomes, trisomy 21, partial trisomy for the short arm, trisomy 18, trisomy 13).

In physiological optics, myopia shows through a focused image in front of the foveal plane).

The higher the myopia, the farther the focal plane is from the retina (Fig. 2.3).

Natural accommodation tends to put this focal plane image away from retina even more. Consequently, and because of not using it, in some myopes, accommodative amplitude is low.

Diverging optic systems, negative in dioptric value, bring the clear image back on the fovea in myopes.

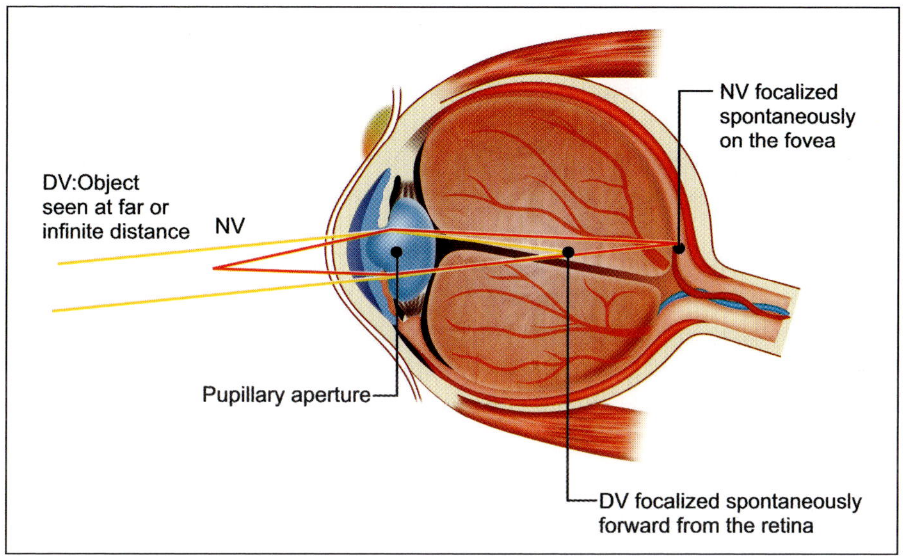

Fig. 2.3 Distant and near vision in optically not compensated myope

In myopes, the focal image in distant vision (DV) projects itself forward from the retina, while the optical image in near vision (NV) projects at the back of it, closer to the fovea according to the degree of ametropia. So much that, without any effort, near vision or very near one is clear for any not compensated myope and presbyopia only leads to a late inconvenience.

We note the myopias by their negative dioptric values:
- low myopia with compensation below –2.00 diopters,
- high myopias beyond –8.00 diopters and,
- moderate myopias in between these values.

    Accommodation cannot compensate myopia for it tends to make it worse.

2.3.2 Childhood Myopia

The discovery of a myopic refraction, with or without cycloplegics, from birth or during childhood is often pathological.

Myopia is liable to evolve with the child's growth.

Cycloplegy is only useful to the myope to exclude the accommodative component.

In order to not overcorrect the subject, as in hyperopia, it is necessary to make out a good exam with blur, as opposed to the use of cycloplegy in children or infants (*See* paragraph 2.2.3, High hyperopia, page 51).

The exam behind refractor being not applicable in children under 5, we will use trial spectacles paying attention to keep only the lowest correction that provides the best visual acuity (*See* paragraph 2.2.4, Optical compensation, page 52).

We will control myopic optical compensation twice a year in case of great evolution (annual increase of 0.50 diopter), or only once a year if relatively stable.

Most of the time, a myopia starting around 6 will evolve, according to its genetical determinism, until 25 to 30 years old. Myopias that appear later are equally subject to evolve later, sometimes after 40 and 45.

Malignant myopias are often high myopias and can get worse until 50 or 60.

2.3.3 Maintaining Near Vision

Compared to early stability of hyperope, myope has a delayed visual tranquility.

Effectively, its optical compensation keeps stable for far vision, but near vision (or very near one) is still good without correction.

As a consequence, when presbyopia comes, myope finds himself taking off his glasses to read and his single vision lens happen to become unsuited to near vision.

We consider near vision between 25 and 50 cm. Beyond 50 cm, we speak about intermediate vision. Below 25 cm, it is very near vision.

As long as the absolute value of the necessary addition to compensate the presbyopia remains inferior to the absolute value of the myopia, the subject can see clearly in near or very near vision without the help of any optical system.

In case of mild myopias superior to –4.00 diopters, presbyopia, fully set in, does not hamper very near vision without optical mediation, even if the working distance is sometimes close and uncomfortable (nose few centimeters away from reading page in high myopias).

In such a situation, myopes physiology allow them to place the near vision image in the foveal plane without accommodative effort, with a sufficient field of vision. This enables the subject to read for hours without strain and explains why so many myopes spontaneously put away their multifocal spectacles for prolonged reading.

Myopes can do without optical correction when they read and keep being concerned about the quality of near vision, whatever the compensation of myopia.

This point is crucial and we will widely debate about it in the next chapter when it will come to choose the most adequate treatment for presbyopia in myopes (*See also* paragraph 3.1.2, Customized spectacles, page 82).

Some particular cases are worth of being mentioned:
- myopic anisometropias (an eye more myope than the other one) or,
- unilateral myopia (one eye is myope, the other one emmetrope).

If abnormality is congenital, patient tolerates the difference between both eyes very well, from a clinical point of view.

It can be different, when one gets abnormality brutally, without any possibility to adapt oneself: visual discomfort close to diplopia because of the aniseikonia.

Aniseikonia is the disparity of an image growth that both eyes see and the ametropia of which is different (anisometropia). An anisometropia superior to 2 diopters is liable to cause aniseikonia, which can show through diplopical phenomena (seeing double objects).

Adaptation of acquired anisometropia is rather awkward, two cases are possible:
- binocular vision can remain. The adaptation capacity of the subject then depends on the subject's level of aniseikonia, on the binocular vision potential and brain plasticity,
- binocular vision cannot be preserved. In the absence of binocular vision, the subject alternates distant image (with near image concomitant neutralization) with near image (with distant image concomitant neutralization) according to his visual needs.

It remains important to make sure our patient has a simple, clear and comfortable vision, in order to preserve his visual needs as much as possible.

Clinical experience proves that congenital myopic anisometropia, when not excessive in dioptric value, and in the absence of amblyopia, represents a true refractive opportunity for the subject who does not know or hardly knows anything about the aftermath of presbyopia, while he or she keeps an excellent far vision.

Patient generally has an alternate vision, all the more since we often discover this type of unilateral myopia rather late.

Myopic eye is "used" in near vision and the emmetropic one in distant vision.

In several cases, these subjects cannot bear any optical correction and live well without binocular vision.

This disposition is so favorable that this anisometropia is, for some people, a refractive model for presbyopia treatment in myopes. We will come to it later (*See also* paragraph 3.3.8, Monovision LASIK, page 108).

In case of amblyopia on the most myopic eye, the situation is less favorable, but remains functionally useful for near vision (relative amblyopic eye).

Amblyopia: Decrease of functional visual results without organic damage. Deep amblyopia is defined by an impaired visual acuity (20/200 or less in distant vision) and opposes relative amblyopia that represents a less serious handicap.

Nonetheless, this situation can happen to be useless, if the myopic eye is deeply amblyopic (less than 20/200 of visual acuity in distant vision).

In this case, presbyope will ask for a near vision apparatus (as emmetropes and other ametropes).

2.4 PRESBYOPIA AND ASTIGMATISMS

Cylindrical ametropias, which we call such a way regarding their optical aerial compensation with the introduction of a cylinder in the correcting lenses, gather the refractive field of the regular astigmatisms.

Spectacles cannot compensate irregular astigmatisms. In regular astigmatisms, there are two main meridians, perpendicular to each other (one curved, one flat).

Etymologically speaking, astigmatism is in relation to, from an optical viewpoint, the fact that the image of a point is not a point but an image interfering with a shade that surrounds the objects we are looking at.

In other words, the refraction varies according to the orientation of the main meridians (orientation with the horizontal defined as the 0°–180° line and the vertical going through 90°) (Fig. 2.4).

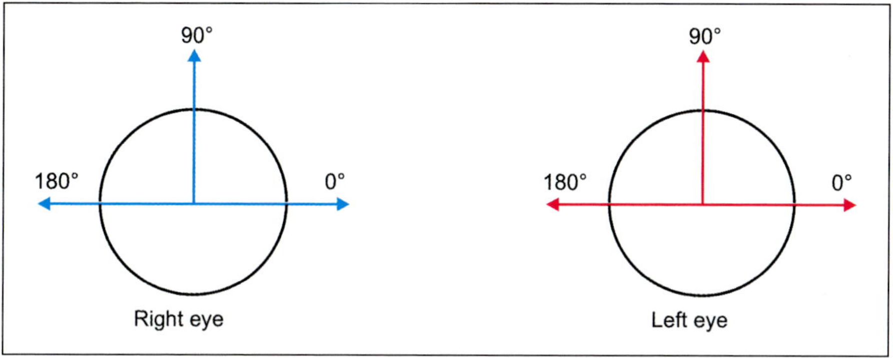

Fig. 2.4 Orientation of meridians according to binasal notation of axis (TABO notation)

2.4.1 Classifications (Fig. 2.5)

Astigmatism is often hereditary with a predominant autosomal transmission, it is then:
- regular (perpendicular axis of astigmatism),
- bilateral,
- often symmetrical (compared to the corneal center),
- with enantiomorphism (mirror orientation of the astigmatism to the sagittal plane).
  Acquired astigmatism may be regular or irregular (two main non-perpendicular meridians).

Acquired regular astigmatisms etiologies are varied, as a consequence of:
- cataract surgery,
- sometimes strabismus,
- retinal detachment,
- ptosis,
- corneal pterygium,
- prolonged wearing of soft or rigid contact lenses (corneal warpage),
- tumor or superior eyelid inflammation,
- senility.

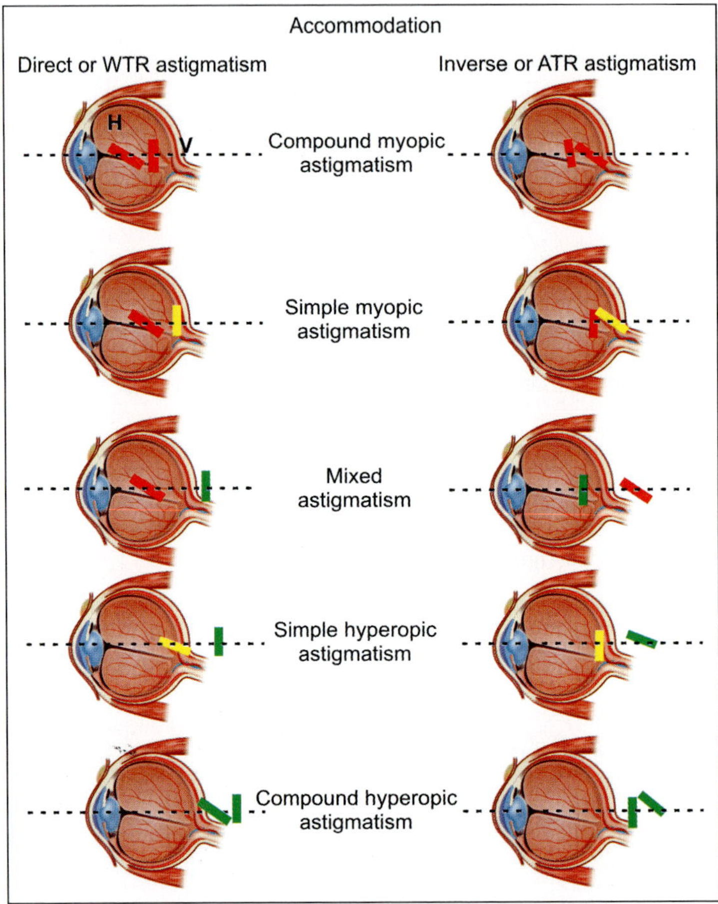

Fig. 2.5 Astigmatism classification

According to the examples of astigmatisms shown hereabove, we see the horizontal image focal (H) corresponding to an object vertical focal is ahead of the vertical focal (V) corresponding to the object horizontal focal. This is the optical disposition of the regular astigmatisms. The myopic focals are in red, the hyperopic focals, in green and the emmetropic ones, in yellow. Direct (respectively indirect) astigmatism is also known as with-the-rule (WTR) astigmatism [respectively against-the-rule (ATR)].

Acquired irregular astigmatisms can:

- coming from the cornea, relate:
  - keratoconus or pellucid marginal degeneration associated with a myopia,
  - traumatically or inflammatory-induced corneal wound healing,
  - degenerative affection or keratosurgery,
- coming from crystalline lens (most often index astigmatism), relate:
  - cataract,
  - coloboma,
  - lenticonus,
  - lenticular ectopia (ectopia lentis),
  - postoperative subluxation of the lens (in particular iridectomy),
- or coming from retina,
- more seldom, relate a posterior staphyloma, a tumor near the posterior pole.

Possible signs coming with them are the accommodative asthenopia, (due to endless fluctuations between the two focal images), the secondary torticoli with inclination of the head that can trigger a scoliosis in children.

We speak about direct astigmatism or with-the-rule (WTR) astigmatism when the vertical meridian is converging more than the horizontal one, inverted astigmatism or against-the-rule (ATR) astigmatism when the horizontal meridian is the most convergent.

Physiologically speaking, the individual can show a certain degree of direct corneal astigmatism that does not exceed 0.75 diopters, which an inverted internal physiological astigmatism generally compensate and does not exceed 0.75 diopters.

Ocular total astigmatism (to be corrected) comes from the association of corneal astigmatism (or external astigmatism) and internal astigmatism (mainly induced by crystalline lens).

We consider the WTR astigmatism as the most frequent and also the best tolerated as far as optics is concerned.

From an optics viewpoint, the splitting of focal images can happen on both images at the front of retinal plane (compound myopic astigmatism), at the back of the foveal plane (compound hyperopic astigmatism), one focal at the front and one focal at the back of retinal plane (mixed astigmatism), or only one split focal on retina, the other one being at the front (simple myopic astigmatism) or at the back of retina (simple hyperopic astigmatism).

2.4.2 Circle of Least Confusion (Fig. 2.6)

From these definitions, an essential optical notion comes in non-compensated astigmats, who naturally look for an optimal vision area between these two focals: the optimal blur circle.

Area of least confusion (or circle of least confusion 'CLC' of the Conoid of Sturm) is connected with a virtual frontal image plane located at "half the segment in diopter" that split the two focal images: that is at a value of C/2 of the two focals, "C" being the value of astigmatism. That is the value of the difference between each of the two main meridians power.

The optimal blur circle comes very close to CLC, but is not always the CLC. If the cylinder is low (inferior to 1.00 diopter), the optimal blur circle can be the CLC; what explains the low astigmats (at least until presbyopia) can do without their astigmatism correction.

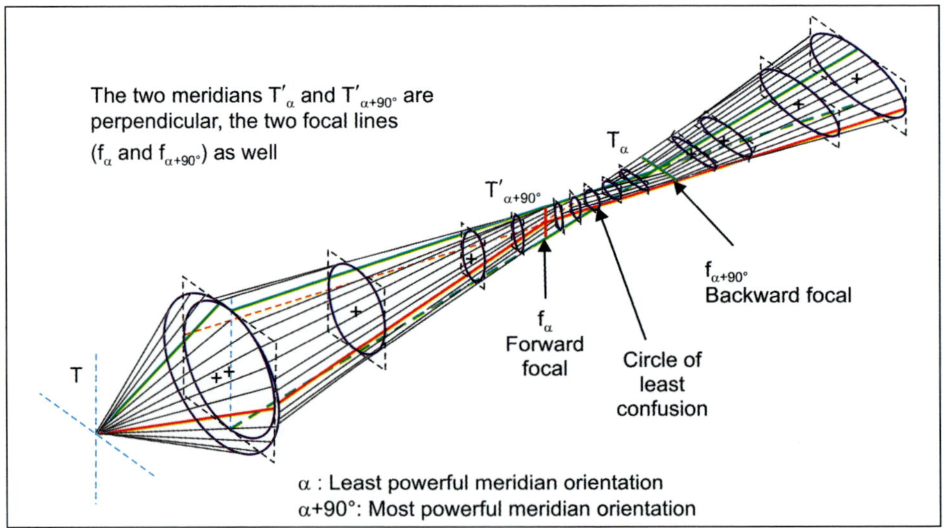

Fig. 2.6 The astigmatic beam

(Excerpt from: "Analyse de la vision: cours d'optique physiologique 1ère année, CLM éditeur.")

Schematically, the entire compensation of astigmatism lies in the optical moving of each focal to bring back on retina.

We can proceed following two distinctive ways:

1. Whether determine the most convex sphere (or the least concave one) giving the best acuity, or the compensatory sphere that corresponds to the least powerful meridian and then determine the power of the compensatory negative cylinder orientated to 90°. Schematically, it would be the same as overlapping the most convergent focal on the least convergent one (taking the focal back is the same as expressing the cylinder in negative algebric value).
2. Or determine the least convex sphere (or the most convex one) giving the best acuity, or the compensatory sphere that corresponds with the most powerful meridian and then determine the compensatory positive cylinder orientated to 90°. Schematically, it would be the same as overlapping the least convergent focal upon the most convergent one (positive cylinder).

In any case, we will have to double check the sphere once we have determined the cylinder power and axis.

We advise to follow the first method for it allows to better control accommodation.

Optical formulas then obtained for astigmats compensation are in spherocylindrical formulas. Getting compensation in negative or positive cylinder must match the same value. We obtain two formulas by transposition from the one to the other.

Example: +2.00 (–3.00)60° formula equivalent to –1.00 (+3.00)150°.

Practitioner uses these equivalent algebric formulas to his liking, but the blurring method being the first we use, we commonly express in negative cylinders (*See* paragraph 2.2.3, High hyperopia, page 51).

What are the characteristic elements of the arrival of presbyopia in astigmats, then? They indeed depend on the type of astigmatism.

2.4.3 Astigmatisms and Accommodation

Troubles that astigmatism induces (headaches, asthenopia, monocular diplopia, photophobia…) depend on the value of ametropia, the age and on the subject himself:

- lack of clearness is more or less conscious,
- confusions among letters or numbers depend on the nature of astigmatism,

- performances of visual acuity can change from an examination to the other, according to the level of fatigue,
- in the cases of simple astigmatism, only cylinder causes a visual trouble; in the cases of compound or mixed astigmatisms, the problems can also be due to the value of the sphere that belongs to the cylinder.

As we noticed earlier (*See* paragraph 2.4.2, Circle of least confusion, page 64), astigmats focus on their optimal blur circle (which can be the circle of least diffusion) as long as they can do it.

By becoming presbyopic, subject feels a discomfort since the blur needs specific accommodation.

We must detect and treat the infant or child suffering from high astigmatism early enough to avoid the onset of a meridian amblyopia (bad vision in certain space orientations).

We can compensate minor astigmatism later, especially at the age of school acquisitions (around 6), because these astigmatisms are particularly penalizing for far vision (black board), much less in near vision (learning reading and writing).

Subjects until around 30 frequently compensate astigmatism, when fall in accommodative performance becomes manifest, with a peculiar trouble in night driving, at the theater, in dark rooms.

It is clear that during tests, decrease in brightness is critical for the thirty-year-old astigmat who then looks for an optical compensation gradually necessary to obtain a good sight.

This is the reason why astigmats rarely wear sunglasses (decrease in brightness increasing the loss of contrast sensitivity), unless adapted to their sight.

2.5 PRESBYOPIA AND OPHTHALMOLOGICAL PATHOLOGIES

As we noticed it above (*See* paragraph 2.4, Presbyopia and astigmatisms, page 60), at varying grades, these non-spherical ametropias can associate with authentical ocular pathologies that modify the perception of presbyopia.

2.5.1 Cataracts

This is the case of the indicial cataracts (induced myopization), which make the patient say, "Doctor, my near vision has been improving awhile, so much that I do not wear my glasses anymore".

We have to remember that onset of nuclear cataract in hyperopes or a hyperopic astigmatism is prone to near vision improvement and reduces the dependence on optical correction. However, this type of cataract worsens myopes or myopic astigmats near vision (smaller and less comfortable reading distance).

Non-indicial cataracts lower near vision without possibility of satisfactory optical compensation (impossible improvement for near visual acuity).

2.5.2 Glaucomas

Glaucomas, which outcome to a constituted optical neuropathy, ordinarily interfere very scarcely with presbyopia since, most often, the central vision remains functional.

It is not the same for the perimetrical form of glaucoma with visible inferior paracentral scotoma or inferior nasal step (impairment of optic nerve superior ganglionic fibers), because the amputation of the inferior visual field has an effect on not only the visibility of the strolling area (stairs, sidewalk, etc.), but also on near vision.

2.5.3 Maculopathies

It is certainly in hereditary maculopathies (Stargardt's disease, Best's disease) or degenerations (ARMD, conus dystrophy) that the trouble in near vision increase the most at the age of presbyopia for accommodation becomes inoperative regarding the more or less utter destruction of the foveolar function.

In such context, and we will talk about it again (*See also* paragraph 3.1.2, Customized spectacles, page 82), an added overcorrection must compensate presbyopia for the enlargement of images, together with a readaptation of visual strategy for the use of fixation secondary retinal foci.

2.5.4 Nystagmus

Nystagmi, whether syndromal (ocular albinism) or isolated, also raise specific problems in near vision when presbyopia appears.

Nystagmus is an oscillatory movement of eyeballs, usually bilateral, horizontal, vertical, oblique or rotatory, of varying amplitude, speed, rhythms, overlapping normal, permanent or intermittent movements.

Nystagmography permits an accurate typing of the nystagmus: direction is given by the quick component.

The pandilar nystagmus is recognizable for its equal and opposed ocular shakes, impression that objects are flickering coming with frequent troubles in accommodation.

The nystagmus of opposed direction to both eyes ("see-saw") is bilateral and asymmetrical, an eye up while the other one goes down, and conversely, in a pandilar manner, more or less in line. In this nystagmus, both eyes have an associate rotatory nystagmus (generally intorsion of the highest eye, extorsion of the lowest one), movement is faster but smaller in the upper look, nystagmus diminishes in near focus or intense light, which allows presbyope to read with a nystagmus.

In case of nystagmus blockade position, we can improve near vision; we will come back to it later concerning antinystagmical surgery and adequate refractive overcorrection (*See also* paragraph 3.1.3, Multifocal lenses, page 84).

2.5.5 Dyslacrima

Chronical lacrimation, by excess of tears or insufficient excretion, and dry syndromes represent major problems for the patients, often elders, suffering from this affection.

A blepharospasm can add up to these troubles and worsen the discomfort in near vision, because, tear film being pathological, then near vision turns out to be hard with trouble issued from the bad legibility through an unstable and irregular lacrymal meniscus lying on the inferior palpebral margin.

2.5.6 Presbyopia and Ocular Aberrations

The modern investigation methods of the sight quality give invaluable help to comprehension and mastery of the ocular aberrations (OA) that can contribute to the improvement of presbyopia compensation.

Sight is a sense including visual envelope. Sensorial vision could not restrict itself to spatial discrimination for it has a usual measure that passes through visual acuity quantitative assessment. It also has abilities more qualitative gathered under the terms of contrast sensitivity, chromatic sense, kinetic sense, and ocular aberrations.

Effectively, these functional evaluation tests are compulsory to customize the approach of ametropias when presbyopia is involved.

These tests must enable:
- an objective evaluation of the effect on life quality (life quality surveys),
- to appreciate the functional troubles that justify an optical compensation (maximum speed reading),
- the follow-up of troubles and their evolution after compensation (contrast sensitivity, accommodation amplitude, binocular vision).

The notion of visual quality (contrast sensitivity, aberrometry) has come to complete the visual quantity (visual acuity): patients may complain while they could read 10/10.

The measure of the ocular aberrations or of all other optical system depends on aberrometry.

2.5.6.1 *Aberrometry* (Fig. 2.7)

The measure of eye's aberrations (aberrometry) allows to quantify optical quality.

These measures have benefited greatly from the Wavefront (WF) clinical application to ocular diopter.

WF is a flat luminous stimulus that undergoes deformations after passing in an imperfect optical system. In an ideally neutral optical system, WF would not undergo any deformation while crossing this system.
Aberrometry analyzes the greatness of the deformations that the incident wavefront has undergone.

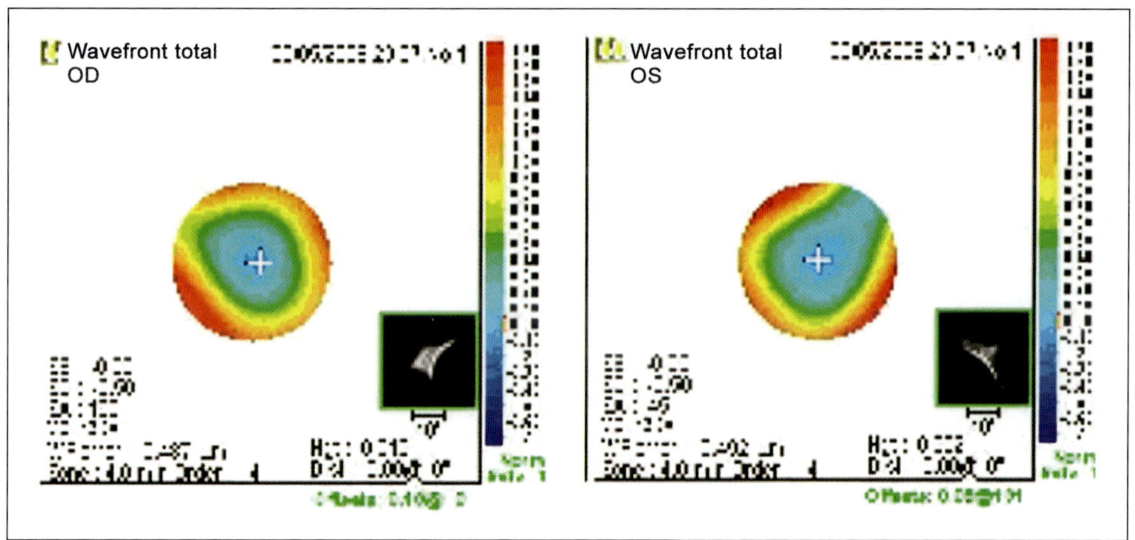

Fig. 2.7 Total aberrometrical profiles in a presbyopic bilateral LASIK postoperative patient. (Personal images obtained on Nidek OPD-scan 10,000 aberrometer)

In this example, the color maps (respectively to the left for the right eye and to the right for the left eye) represent the total aberrometrical profiles (total wavefront). These maps translate the deformation of a wavefront (WF), which covers all ocular transparent media (cornea, anterior chamber, crystalline lens, vitreous). Here, green corresponds, on the colorimetric scale, to the absence of wavefront deformation. "Warmer" colors show a wavefront lead, whereas cold colors show a delay. Broadly speaking, the error of the total wavefront is the same on the left eye (0.192 μm deviation) and on the right eye (0.187 μm), in this example.

Wavefront (WF) technology made possible to send of a homogeneous luminous beam in the patient's eye and thus to receive he optical ocular aberrations (OA) coming back from ocular transparent interfaces.

We classify the OA by level in ascending order:
- the aberrations of low level being elementary (spherocylindrical correction),
- High order aberrations (HOA) are thinner and more subtle (spherical aberration, coma, triangular or quadrangular astigmatism).

OA, after mathematical analysis, come down to an algebrical sum of Zernicke polynomials (Z) or Fourier transform.

We could say the mathematical approach by Fourier transform is significantly more accurate than Z expansion, although we commonly use the latter to work out the of WF data.

We can then write Z polynomials as a sum of coefficients "Z" with an exponent representing the aberration's order level (n), and a dashdotted function for spatial frequency (m): Z (m, n).

Eye can have refraction troubles: Myopia or hyperopia (defocusing) and astigmatism that are level 2 aberrations, level 1 aberrations having no clinical correlation.

OA (Fig. 2.8) are then classified in ascending order according to their type, and we describe HOA (n superior to 2) that have a clinical expression as follows:
- comas (level n = 3),
- triangular astigmatisms (level n = 3) or,
- quadrangular astigmatism (level n = 4),
- spherical aberration (level n = 4).

Amongst OA of low and high orders, we also mention spatial frequency (m) in order to classify them:
- frequency is nul (m = 0) with non-repetitive OA, meaning morphology with a rotational symmetry in space (defocusing, spherical aberration),
- when symmetry axis, frequency is called unique (comas m = 1),
- when pattern repeated twice, three or four times, frequency is respectively double (m = 2), triple (m = 3) or quadruple (m = 4).

There are HOA of a level even superior, but they have a slight clinical interest (residual value).

Here are some examples of Zernicke monomials with their denominations:
- Z_{-2}^{2} = inverted astigmatism,
- Z_{0}^{2} = myopic or hypermetropic defocusing,

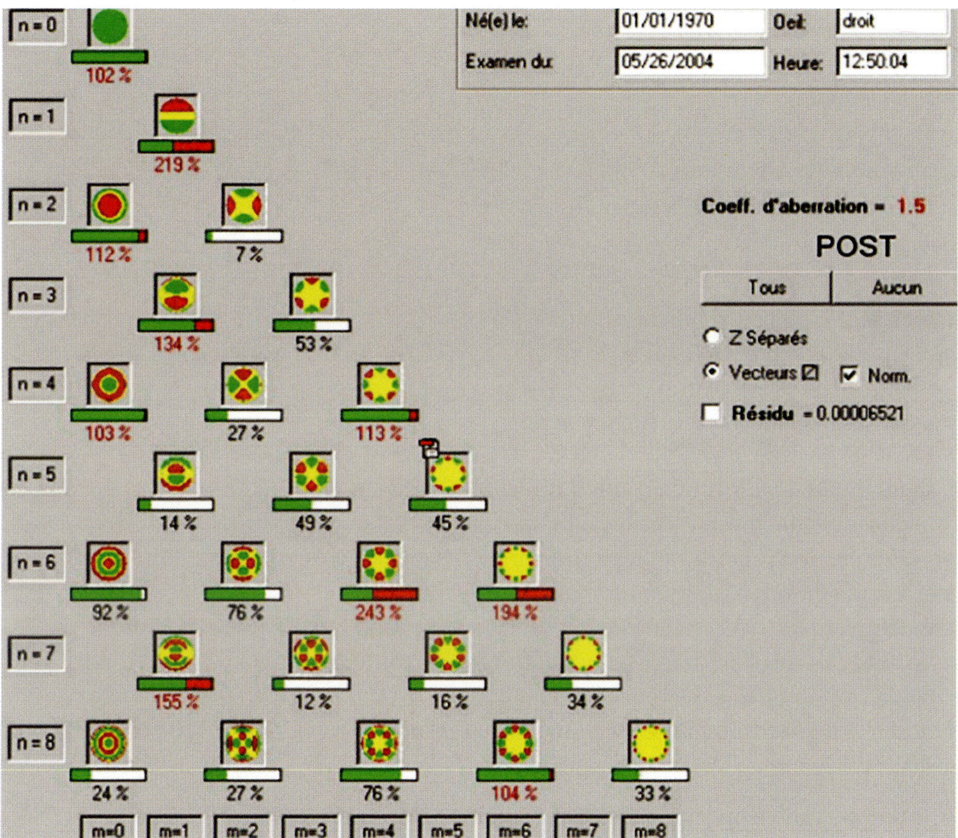

Fig. 2.8 Corneal aberrometry example to the 8th order (HR Pentacam)
(Digital image taken out from an anterior segment analyzer Pentacam type)

In this example, OA are sorted from lowest (n = 0) to high 8th order level (n = 8) on y-axis. On x-axis are the special frequencies of the different aberrations studied (m). Each aberration is modelized in miniature and relative range is expressed in percentage. When OA is physiologically excessive, over epression is marked in red with the corresponding percentage. It is the case of direct coma (Z_1^3) identified with 134% from normality, total OA sum being 1.5 aberration coefficient, since HOA beyond the 8th order level are insignificant (residual value=6.10^{-5}).

- Z_2^2 = direct astigmatism,
- Z_{-3}^3 = inverted triangular astigmatism,
- Z_{-1}^3 = inverted coma,
- Z_1^3 = direct coma,
- Z_3^3 = direct triangular astigmatism,
- Z_4^4 = inverted quadrangular astigmatism,
- Z_{-2}^4 = inverted quadrangular astigmatism,
- Z_0^4 = spherical aberration,
- Z_2^4 = direct quadrangular astigmatism,
- Z_{-3}^4 = direct quadrangular astigmatism.

Total aberrometry is the sum of these different terms.

There are mathematical formulas with a direct or positive phase (+) for each type of OA (a sinusoid describes the phase) or the inverse phase (–) that a cosine function describes.

We then describe each aberration with the symbol Z (for Zernicke, the first to describe OA polynomial formula): dash-dotted level (n), frequential row (m) as exponent.

This way, complete eye OA come down to the polynomial addition of all Z elements.

Each term expresses itself in Root-Mean-Square (RMS) of micrometrical
WF deviation compared to a reference plane (Fig. 2.9).

WF, after penetration through the eye, may be early (positive values), in the plane (nil value) or late (negative value), compared to the reference plane.

Aberrometric may be shown on tridimensional graphic or colorimetric flat projection:
- *red*: front's lead,
- *green*: front in the plane,
- *blue*: front's delay.

All the OA are widely spread among as much the healthy subjects as the subjects with visual troubles. It is only their greatness and their evolution in time that give the vision bad quantity and quality.

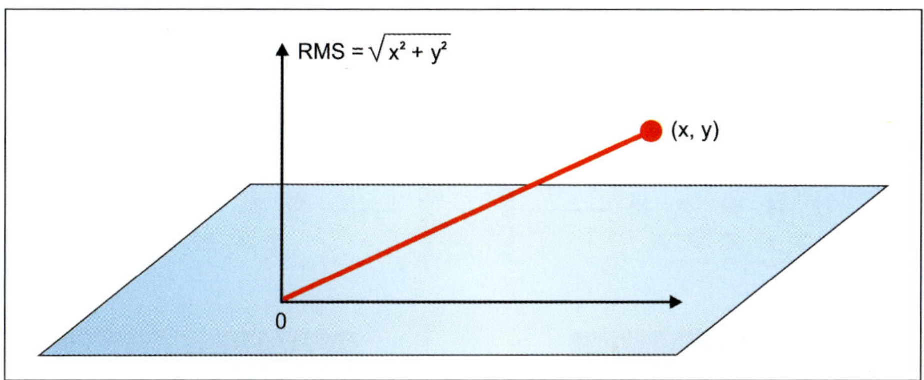

Fig. 2.9 Spatial representation of WF deviation under RMS form

Every aberrometric term proves clinical lesion of uneven extent. Thus, usual spherocylindrical corrections compensate both defocusing and astigmatism: the subjective discomfort is well known (visual blur, contours or shade imperfection).

Conversely, comas show through a blur in a trail effect as seen advanced keratoconus (vertical coma).

Comatic clinical expression consists usually of a bad sight or a monocular diplopia, without too much complaint in night conditions. This is even more the case since the coma value reaches or exceeds 1.00 µm in RMS value.

However, small value of coma can be necessary: this is what we meet in some supervision cases.

We widely observe triangular astigmatisms Z_3^3 and quadrangular astigmatism Z_{-2}^4 in keratoconic subjects.

2.5.6.2 Spherical Aberrations

The spherical aberrations Z_0^4 lead to visual discomfort in mesopic and scotopic condition (halos, blur) impairing essentially night driving (Fig. 2.10).

Tridimensional representation looks such as a Mexican "sombrero": the more the aspect is symmetrical, the purer the OA.

All optical spherical surfaces show spherical aberrations linked with fact that central beams do not refract as in the periphery.

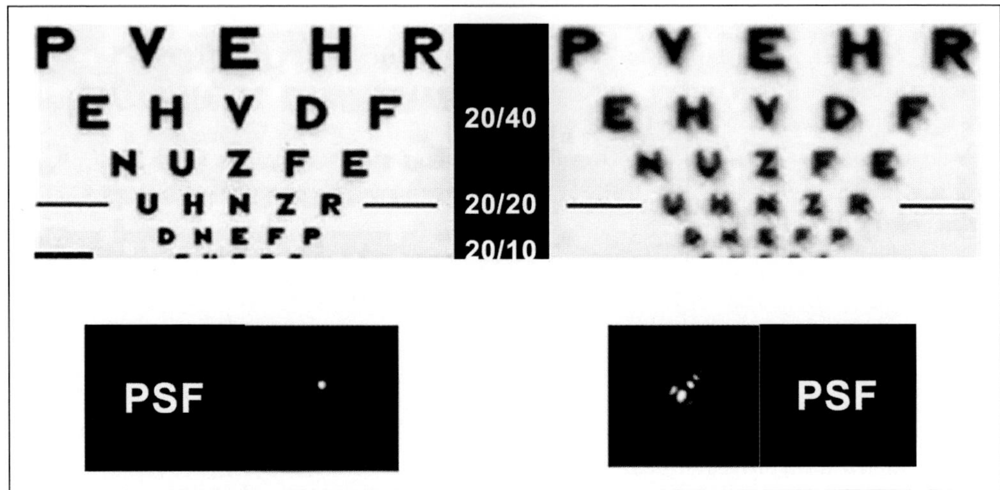

Fig. 2.10 Point spread function (PSF) and aberropic visual simulation

Visual simulation allows to identify loss in visual quality for a 3-mm diameter pupil:

- on the left for emmetropic eye without aberropia (20/20 corresponds to the horizontal line),
- on the right for eye affected with low level OA (myopia) and HOA (spherical aberrations).

On the right, a point is seen without deformation while on the left the same point is seen with some spreading (PSF).

Proportionally to their optical power, cornea, natural crystalline lens, IOLs are likely to generate spherical aberrations.

In young subjects, corneal negative spherical aberrations (corneal curvature higher in the center then in the periphery) naturally compensate crystalline lens positive spherical aberrations (peripheral beams more refracted than central beams).

With the coming of presbyopia and after, crystalline lens alters. It does not compensate corneal aberrations anymore, and the system produces positive spherical aberrations.

Brimonidine with myotic action may give functional results in this type of trouble with a 0.24 mm to 0.50 mm reduced pupil in day light and prevention for mydriasis at night.

The so-called "normal" human eye presents, in small proportions, a mixture of OA.

OA vary in time (accommodation) and in space (pupil size), so much that aberrometers (according to Hartmann-Schack, Tscherning or skiascopical principle) only scarcely give exactly identical values except under cycloplegics (*See also* paragraph 1.3.4, Accommodative insufficiencies, page 15).

This demonstrates the extreme sensitivity of instrumental measures, hence difficulty to determine the border between physiological state and optical abnormality to be compensated.

We estimate the relative involvement of OA in vision impairment as follows:
- defocusing and primary astgmatism (70%),
- coma (10%),
- spherical aberration (15%),
- the other abnormalities counting for less than 5% effects on vision (residual errors).

2.5.6.3 Multifocal WF

The WF aberrometry enables the quantification and qualification of ocular multifocality taking into account:
- the relationship between refraction and pupillometry (*See also* paragraph 1.3.2, Miosis, page 13),
- the cartography of this multifocality,
- the coefficients of HOA interfering with the nature of this multifocality (spherical aberration, coma).

The modulation transfer functions (MTF) gathers the capacity of the optical system to transmit contrasts. We can express them whether in a simulated image of an optotype or an object as seen, or in a modelization of the light beams.

The point spread function (PSF) also gives an idea about the quality of the vision in two dimensions (*See* Fig. 2.6).

We can simulate the sensitivity to contrast by means of contrast sensitivity function (CSF) and quantify on a bar graph to appreciate sensitivity to different contrasts (usually 10%, 20%, 100% and average).

Adaptative optics (AO) enables to real-time connection between visual strategy and OA.

The AO is a scientific discipline to control OA of system. Aberrometric analysis allows the conception of an optical masking counter-system to reduce or cancel all or part of various observed OA.

We can assess sensitivity to dazzle classically with the functional recovery curve or more recently thanks to the brain activity analysis with functional magnetic resonance imaging (MRI).

Positive spherical aberration and coma are HOA, which produce by themselves natural multifocality favorable to presbyopia.

In distant vision (relative mydriasis), positive and negative spherical aberrations are unfavorable. In near vision (relative miosis), negative spherical aberration is favorable, while the positive one is unfavorable for presbyopia.

In hyperopes and emmetropes, presbyopia is increased with a narrow pupil, because near vision is penalized during accommodation-convergence-miosis synkinesis (*See also* paragraph 1.3.1, Synkinesis, page 12).

Natural direct comatic aberration shares the eye optic diaphragm in two zones: a superior one for distant vision, and an inferior one for near vision. It then enables a partial compensation of presbyopia.

Accommodative dynamic generates OA owing to near vision, like negative spherical aberration and coma.

Apart from spherocylindrical ametropias, some authors called aberropia visual impairment due to HOA.

Aberropia would then result from a global negative effect linked with HOA, whether stemming from an inadequacy between favorable and unfavorable aberrations or caused by unfavorable aberrations, what comes together with an impairment of the visual performance.

To correct aberropia, as a refractive error, positive and negative OA may interact with each other.

Even more recently, AO contributed to the study of human optical imperfections. When applied to ophthalmology, AO technology contributed to correct, even to adjust HOA so as to better understand effects on human vision.

In ophthalmology, AO is considered as a sophisticated technique that allows to correct or adjust the rate of HOA of the ocular WF.

Correction of low and high OA with an AO device can theoretically give the eye, in monochromatic light, an optical quality limited by only diffraction.

In these conditions, relationships between the dimensions of diffraction focal spot and foveal photoreceptor diameter condition the ocular discrimination.

The AO confirm supervision ability in accordance with experimental conditions: retinal illuminance diameter, in the absence of OA, to be estimated to 3 µm (for a pupillary diameter of 6 mm and a focal length of 20 mm), this maximum resolution corresponding with a visual acuity of around 20/40.

Moreover, AO has made possible study of the adaptation mechanism, from neurovisual system to the OA: AO enable to correct HOA, but also AO can modulate it. Thus HOA may provide potentially beneficial effects (multifocality induction).

Training in the neurovisual system facilitates compensation, even partially, of the visual blur brought by permanent OA.

After review about ametropias and ophthalmological pathologies that influence presbyopia and vice versa, we are now going to take interest in the possible optical compensations of presbyopia.

2.5.6.4 Quality of Vision

Modern investigation methods about vision quality are precious help to understand and control ocular aberrations (OA) which contribute to improve presbyopia compensation.

Sight is a sense contained in the so-called visual envelope. The sensorial vision could not limit itself to spatial discrimination since its routine measurement is based on the quantitative evaluation of visual acuity. It also has more quantitative aptitudes such as contrast sensitivity, chromatic sense, kinetic sense, and, more recently reported, OA.

Indeed, the importance of these functional evaluation tests is paramount if we want to customize ametropic approach at the time of presbyopia.

These tests ought to allow:
- objective assessment of the impact on the quality of life (quality of life survey),
- to appreciate functional troubles that justify an optical compensation (maximum reading speed),
- awareness of troubles felt and their evolution after compensation (contrast sensitivity, accommodative amplitude, binocular vision).

Notion of visual quality (contrast sensitivity, aberrometry) has come to complete visual quantity (visual acuity) from the time when some operated patients complained despite their 20/20 reading.

The measurement of OA depends on aberrometry.

2.5.6.5 *Corneal Asphericity and OA*

If cornea were spherical, the rate of HOA would be so important that images projected on the retina would be deprived of all visual quality.

In normal population, we know that 80% of corneas are prolate, meaning aspherical, with a mean Q value of –0.26.

Keratometry shows this multifocality with the corneal center arching more than the flatter periphery.

As plotted in average population, cornea has a positive spherical aberration ($Z(n = 4, m = 0)$) of +0.23 µm, crystalline lens a negative spherical aberration of –0.16 µm.

If accommodation enables visual acuity, it seems that, during accommodative process, total spherical aberration compensation provides visual quality.

Accommodative phenomenon induces a dynamic change in HOA direction (coma and spherical aberration).

From the optical point of view, imbalance in corneal and internal spherical aberration rate leads to a bad compensation of OA.

Physiological hyperopization with aging results in a modification of corneal sphericity factor that strives for a sphere and thus increases positive spherical aberrations rate of this sphere.

Aberrometrical study demonstrates that with time crystalline lens reduces negative asphericity without necessarily becoming positive.

CHAPTER 3

Presbyopia and Optical Compensations

Notion of optical *compensation* is particularly adequate to the field of presbyopic care. Indeed, at the moment, refractive ophthalmologist can advise his patient about compensation with:

- spectacle correction,
- precorneal contact lenses,
- or refractive surgery interventions.

Compensation is a temporary palliative treatment, to reappraise periodically and which we cannot consider as a curative treatment.

In most cases, presbyopia compensation:

- precipitates primary prevention (appearance of the affection),
- does not hamper neither secondary prevention (worsening of the affection),
- nor tertiary prevention (appearance of some presbyopic complications).

Optical compensation becomes necessary when the patient feels a marked, permanent, disabling or handicapping trouble for his professional or personal activities.

Early retired and retired themselves have considerably increased their demands standard over these last decades.

Middle-aged patients, still have plenty of activities and passions to satisfy in several occupations: strolling, running, hiking, traveling, reading, bridge playing, crosswords, sewing, doing embroidery, internet, etc. Their visual expectation covers a large field from near vision to distance.

Optical compensation experience actually depends on the individual psychological profile, and on determination of a possible pre-existing ametropia.

Presbyopic subject has an even harder time to adapt to the need for a correction at all times as a help for intermediate or near vision, all the more since he has never had any optical compensation before (emmetropes, low hyperopes).

Use of microcomputer within middle-aged generation and beyond has revealed many micropathologies that were not troublesome until then: microstrabismi, accommodative asthenopia.

Work on microcomputer requires, when presbyopic age comes, adaptation to intermediate vision optical compensation (one arm length reading distance, what compels to take into account prolonged intermediate working distance, added to the near one (reading, knitting...) and the distant one (driving, TV, cinema...) in the majority of our patients.

In the old days, visual specificities in intermediate vision only concerned a limited number of presbyopes: musicians, draftsmen...

3.1 PRESBYOPIA AND SPECTACLES

We commonly call spectacles some ophthalmic lenses that are adapted on adequate frame.

Optical compensation is aerial when in the surrounding air. It is called we call it (sub) aquatical for a using of ophthalmic lenses in specific areas (diving mask, swimming goggles).

3.1.1 Addition Determining

Prior to any determination of near vision addition value, the subject must provide himself with the more convex compensation for distant vision: subjective monocular check, biocular balance and binocular accommodative relaxation examination.

We will appreciate relative comfort in distant vision at the end of the entire visual examination. This, in order to take the appropriate decision in the prescription.

3.1.1.1 With Maximum Accommodation Research

Once maximum accommodation determined (*See also* paragraph 1.4.3.1, Search for maximal accommodation, page 21), we divide this value by two-thirds; what gives us theoretical comfortable accommodation:

$$\text{Theorical comfortable accommodation} = \text{maximum accommodation} \times \frac{2}{3}$$

Then we determine addition according to the working usual distance "d":

$$\text{Add} = \frac{1}{d} - \text{comfortable accommodation.}$$

3.1.1.2 *With a Duochrome Test (See also Figs 1.8 and 1.9)*

The principle of this test is coming from the eye's longitudinal chromatic aberrations (*See also* paragraph 1.4.3.2, Duochrome test, page 22), and it may then be inadequate in certain pathologies, and in certain subjects.

The patient gets his convex maximal compensation in distant vision with trial frame, equipped with addition binocularly or estimated addition according to the age.

We set Duochrome test at the patient usual working distance:
- if patient sees more contrasted in the green area: add positive spheres binocularly, until obtaining contrast equality between optotypes perception in both red and green zones,
- if patient sees more contrasted in the red area: add negative spheres binocularly, until obtaining contrast equality between optotypes perception in both red and green zones,
- if contrast equality between optotypes perception in both red and green zones, addition is correct.

3.1.1.3 *With a Jackson's Cross-cylinder Test (See also Fig. 1.11)*

This test is used with a refractor: we binocularly add a fixed cross-cylinder (FCC) to patient with convex maximal compensation in distant vision, and addition worn or estimated according to the age.

With the FCC +0.50 (−1.00) 90°, we induce a direct astigmatism superimposed on worn correction. This method can then be inadequate in high astigmatism, as well as in patients presenting with non-compensated low astigmatism.

We put the Jackson's cross at usual working distance:
- if patient sees more contrasted in the horizontals: add positive spheres binocularly, until obtaining equal contrast between perception in both horizontals and verticals,
- if patient experiences more contrasted vision in the verticals: add negative spheres binocularly, until obtaining equal contrast between perception in both horizontals and verticals,
- if equality in both verticals and horizontals contrast; the addition is correct.

Whatever the method, test compensation with trial frame, trying to respect, as much as possible, usual working conditions (distance, light, position...).

For working distance of 40 cm, addition should not exceed +2.50 diopters (+3.00 to 33 cm). Nevertheless, if subject works at a peculiar distance, or in case of amblyopic, additions can be higher.

3.1.2 Customized Spectacles (Fig. 3.1)

The customization of glasses and frame seems essential to all professionals of vision.

Technical constraints must be able to adapt to the way of using spectacles (sports, sedentary profession, accountancy), according to the position of heads and visual strategy (stiff neck, cervical spondylosis, visionaute or cephalonaute).[3]

The lenses of presbyopic subject must allow to adapt vision in different light conditions:

- in scotopic condition: white glasses with antiglare treatments, with possibly an antistatic treatment to limit dirtying,
- glasses not exceeding the ANSI standard transmittance category 1 for vision in mesopic luminous condition,
- finally, solar tainted or polarizing glasses, with a color adapted according to the type of activity and/or visual comfort.

Frames must be curved for an efficient protection against UV-rays in photopic light.

In presbyopes, we must painstakingly determine the optical compensation:

- hyperope must have maximal convex compensation in distant vision when presbyopia arrives, if he can bear it,
- myope can possibly be under-corrected to delay the wearing of multifocal glasses, if he wants it and if he can bear such a correction.

When presbyopia comes, need for correction in distant, intermediate and near vision implies forgetting unifocal glasses to use multifocals:

- as one can expect, we determine unifocal glass, for a given visual distance, the depth of field will depend on accommodative reserve,

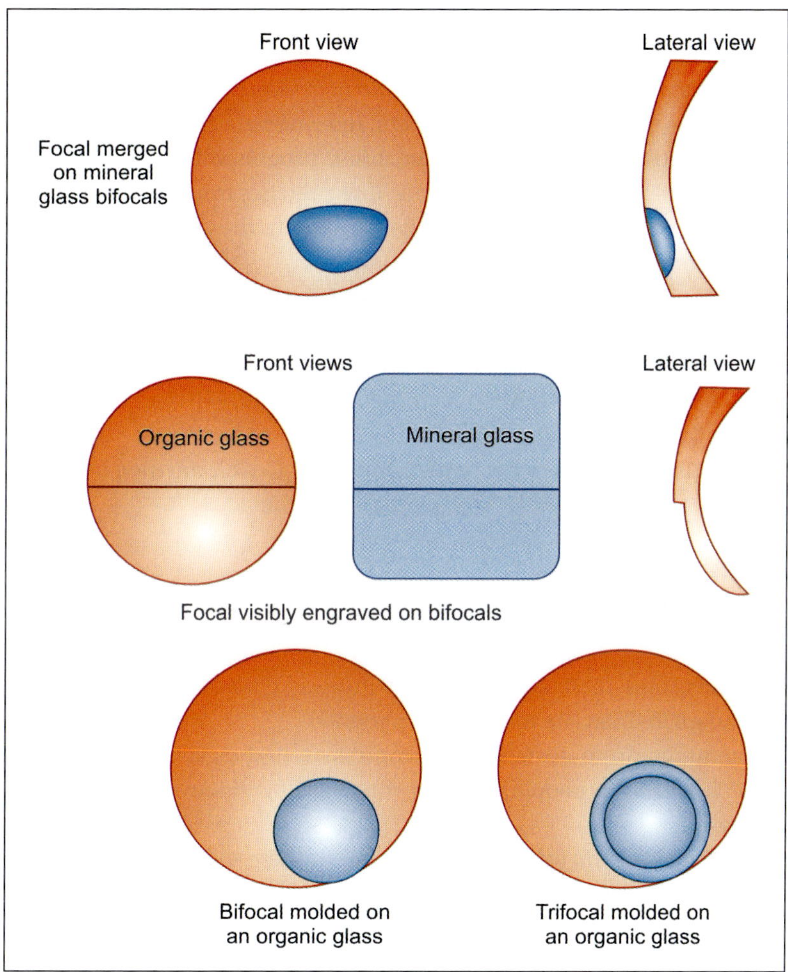

Fig. 3.1 Examples of bifocal and trifocal glasses

- bifocal glass detains two tracks of vision: distant vision and near vision (with an additional chip); or for some particular equipment, distant vision and intermediate one (in this case, arrange for large segment dedicated to intermediate vision) or intermediate and near vision,
- the trifocal glass contains three vision tracks: distant, intermediate and near vision,
- multifocal lens, or progressive lens, shows controlled progression of additive power that we have determined with addition in near vision. Its vision zone stretches from distant to near vision, and
- semi-progressive lens, or proximity lens, shows decrease from the compensating power in near vision. Vision zone stretches from near to intermediate vision.

In office environment, proximity lens enables intermediate vision at the top of the lens, and near vision at the bottom. This spectacle has to be taken off for distant vision and especially interests the patients who prefer, for comfort or specific ametropia, not to wear any correction in distant vision.

The more presbyopia, the more the addition increases. As a result, gap rises between distant vision in the upper part of the glass and near vision in lower part.

This is why we advise presbyopic patients in their fifties not to wait too long before they try progressive glass spectacles. It indeed facilitates comfort and adaptation to them.

3.1.3 Multifocal Lenses

French optics industry has applied for many patents regarding multifocal lenses. It has imposed itself in Europe in progressive lens field, just as the Germans have.

And yet, there remains some reluctance to change unifocal glasses to get progressive ones, due to the persisting difficulty to adapt to them (up to 5% of the patients).

Signs are mostly stemming from destabilizing progression in the glass: difficulty to locate the steps of stairs (causing frequent falls in elder people), neither practical for window-watching, nor easy for handymen (hard to work on ceiling).

Prefer optician who listens to you carefully, and do not hesitate to mention both how you will use your spectacles and all specific activities you are supposed do.

When optician delivers new spectacles, he should explain the good use of the glasses and the precautions to take regarding geometry.

Nonetheless, upscale progressive lenses only satisfy the wide majority of users under few conditions:
- relevant choice for frame, the optician is there to advise you,

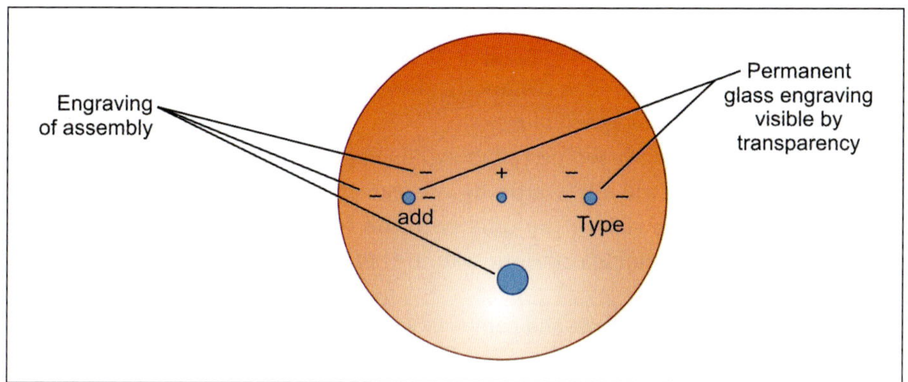

Fig. 3.2 Example of progressive glass

- glass geometry must be in adequacy with the use of the patient,
- if the patient is already wearing progressive spectacles and satisfied with it, go for the same type of geometry,
- although entry-level glasses are cheaper, they are not adapted to all presbyopes,
- we must take the measurements thoroughly. Progressive lenses (Fig. 3.2) centering is essential in presbyopes who have to be able to use different available vision tracks in the glass with minimal gesture and optimal ease,
- distant compensation must be as convex as possible (according to the patient's visual comfort) and addition must not be too high. For the great majority of presbyopes, addition is coherent regarding the age.

It is still too often that we find too high additions, leading to undercompensated hyperopias (not "positive" enough distant vision) or overcompensated myopias (too "negative" distant vision). This remains a well known cause of progressive lenses rejections:

- inappropriate correction of small cylinders. Before prescribing a cylinder of 0.25 or 0.50 diopter to a subject who has ever worn any astigmatism correction, we should make sure there is a real benefit from this correction:
  - visual acuity gain thanks to cylinder and not to spherical equivalent,

- increased visual comfort thanks to cylinder,
- it is not about any tensional astigmatism (generally inverted or oblique).

Otherwise, distortions that the eye-lens distance induces would happen to be particularly disturbing, even more in case of progressive glass spectacles.

Besides, unless really beneficial, we would rather avoid changing power and/or cylinder axis just before first progressive lenses. Then and even afterwards, be aware to all variations of astigmatism:

- we should also test binocular vision: the quality of the fusion and stereoscopic vision. In case of abnormalities, if possible, do suitable orthoptic training before making any eyeglasses.

Binocular vision is normal if clear and simple and comfortable. Binocular vision is abnormal if double, blurred or uncomfortable (related to symptoms).

We have considered for a long time that anisometropic patients, and deprived from binocular vision, could not wear progressive or digressive glasses; this is not exactly right.

Even though these cases remain the most frequent causes for patients not adapting to progressive glass, majority of them get used to it without any problem.

The marks of dirt and other traces remaining on ophthalmic glass often annoy presbyopes a lot. We have to be convincing about the importance of choosing good quality treatments for glass surface, associated with antistatic treatment.

It is widely accepted that cleaning the glasses of spectacles again and again with detergents as stain remover or household products may alter irreversibly optical surface. Please, keep off these products from your spectacles.

To take care of glasses, we have to use specific products or a clean chamois wipes, to avoid wiping glasses with any tissue, for it could scratch them, and to alter surface treatment. So we protect treatments and synthetic glass, not expose spectacles to high heat (do not leave them in car parked in full sun, do not wear them in sauna or hammam…).

In case of intolerance to progressive glasses, your ophthalmologist will take care to check optical quality (entry, middle or high end), which some optician partners scarcely put into question, and to check the absence of all binocular vision abnormalities.

The discovery of decompensated horizontal heterophoria can lead to ad hoc orthoptic rehabilitation.

Heterophoria or dysphoria is a convergence disparity between both eyes by oculomuscular dysfunction. Trouble is often latent, examined with cover-test. Heterophoria can be in convergence (esophoria) or in divergence (exophoria).

Just as in case of vertical heterophorias, after 4 or 5 years of re-education, recurrent decompensation in horizontals would lead to prescribe prismation included in the ophthalmic glass.

Heterophoria or phoria or dysphoria defines the position of the eyes in passive position, fusion is utterly dissociated. Phoria is said "decompensated" when the subject cannot keep fusion comfortable: binocular vision can then be blurred or split; complaints of headaches, ocular itching or burning-sensation, eyestrain excessive lacrymation…

It is more and more frequent that a convergence default, resistant to orthoptics rehabilitation, unveils a postural impairment syndrome (dysproprioception).[4]

The proprioception is the sense of body segments (*See also* paragraph 1.4.2, Ergonomics, page 20). This direction plays a part in statics (orthostatism) and dynamics (running, jumping, etc.). Proprioception clinical pathways interest several organs:
- feet, eyes,
- teguments (skin),
- internal ear, jaws,
- vestibular system, and
- musculoskeleton.

An impairment of this sense (dysproprioception) leads to involuntary and unconscious phenomenon. Compensative phenomenon sometimes induces pains, contractures or vertigos.

In clinical posturology, proprioceptive deficiency is within the range of multimodal therapeutic approach. At ophthalmoposturological level, oculomotor stimulation is based on the interposition of low power prisms, which balance the visual adaptation (active prismation).

Re-equilibration must come with a rehabilitation possibly in association with the other captors (proprioceptive soles, orthognathic splint, orthopraxis, vestibular rehabilitation) in order to make out a global postural reprogrammation.

Decompensated ocular dysproprioception comes with a tonical contracture of trunk, neck musculature and oculomotor muscles influencing presbyopic incomfort with progressive lenses spectacles.

As long as a subject does not compensate dysproprioception, progressive spectacles may be not well tolerated.

This is, in my opinion, a frequent and curable cause of intolerance to progressive glasses that we have to take into account, instead of proposing an optical compensation with bifocal glasses, less esthetic and less functional, or even two different pairs of spectacles.

How technical optic glasses adaptation may be, even with the most recent progressive lenses, presbyopic patient can ask for an occasional contactological solution (as a complement of his spectacles) or permanent (replacing his spectacles).

3.2 PRESBYOPIA AND CONTACT LENSES

As all precorneal lenses, adaptation in contact lenses needs taking into account different factors in order to improve handling, comfort and duration of wearing.

In presbyopes asking for occasional lenses, the best choice will be to go for hydrophilic soft contact lenses: disposable, hydrogel or silicohydrogel ones.

The appearance of soft lenses on the market (until then hydrogel) with variable silicone content enabled a widening of the offer to wearers:
- prolonged wearing made possible with a permeability superior to oxygen,
- better tolerance on dry eyes because of lower hydrophilia.

Silicohydrogel soft lenses are more resistant by touch and sometimes give the impression of a certain adhesion on the eye, in spite of their high permeability to oxygen that allows a more or less prolonged wearing during night and day.

3.2.1 Soft Lenses (Fig. 3.3)

The presbyope adaptation with contact lenses must take into account patient activities (golf, nautism, aerial sports, work conditions, handling of the lenses on a responsibility post).

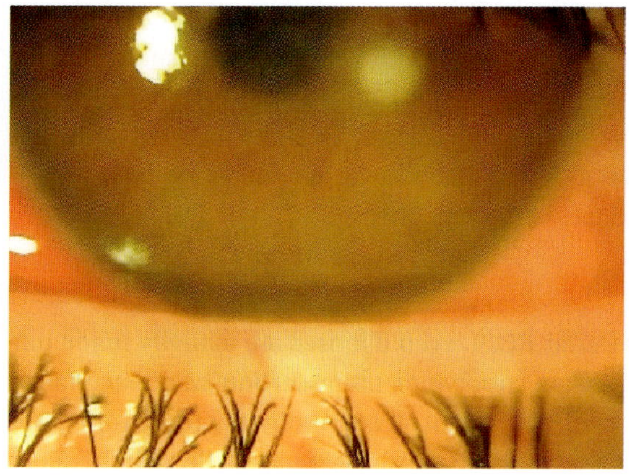

Fig. 3.3 Corneal abscess developed under contact lens (Personal picture obtained on digital RO5000 Rodenstock slit lamp)

The abscess (white disk) under precorneal contact lens is a scarce but severe contactological complication. Indeed, it can lead to eye perforation or corneal wound with visual artefacts. Like anyone wearing contact lenses, presbyope with lenses must respect recommended hygiene, handling and care rules, and should consult a doctor in case of the slightest doubt. Early and well-targeted treatment is often the most efficient.

Disposable contact lenses: one-day, one-week, 15-day, 1-month or 3-month use lenses will be to replace presbyopic spectacles.

In the presence of greasy tears soiling lenses, short-term disposable contact lenses will fit best, as opposed to asymptomatical and very tolerant people who will be up for longer term disposable contacts.

In case of initial adaptation, lenses handling can dissuade the presbyope, even more when he has not put on his first lens and when the subject is not able to see correctly without his spectacles!

Contrary to teenagers, presbyopes using lenses are far more worried about hygiene, as the low rate of infections under contact lenses in this age bracket shows it (Fig. 3.3).

Detailed information and care notebook will be part of the meticulous education of wearers.

It is always important to remind patients of hygiene rules (clean and dry hands, exclusive use of rinsing products, disposing of the lenses if any doubt, frequent deproteinization) to avoid all surface infection (abscess under lens, amibian keratitis) (Fig. 3.3).

We have to exclude all received ideas about the impossibility for presbyopes to wear lenses, especially in high ametropic, astigmats and anisometropes.

Contactological solutions do exist and we should propose them to all the presbyopes who ask for them.

And yet, some optical compensatory solutions do exist, too, and for all age brackets and all types of ametropias, spherical or not, as we are about to see it (*See also* paragraph 3.2.3, Principles of contact lenses adaptation, page 90).

Presbyopic patient chooses between soft lenses, more or less hydrophilic according to the material used, and rigid contact lenses permeable to oxygen. Last years, soft lenses in hydrogel silicone have claimed the high gas permeability, property reserved to rigid contact lenses up to now.

3.2.2 Hard Contact Lenses

By using the adjective "rigid", patients may be reluctant to wear RGPL even if lenses are actually made out of semi-rigid materials (siloxane styrene and fluoromethacrylate copolymer, fluorocarbon-silico- acrylates, Boston XO); while soft contact lenses remain favorable among a market of all age, including presbyopic.

The experience in contactology does not counter completely this first impression, even though the most motivated patients better and better may keep the rigid gas permeable lenses (RGPL).

Then why continue to propose RGPL? You may wonder. Because RGPL is the first choice for presbyopes with high corneal astigmatisms (internal toric hard lens) or total (external toric hard lens), due to:
- refractive stability,
- the low rate of infectious complication,
- the ability of wearing night and day over a period of a month,
- and the quality of follow-up in people wearing RGPL (some patients have been wearing them for 45 years without any inconvenience).

3.2.3 Principles of Contact Lenses Adaptation

Soft contact lenses (SCL) have got the advantage of offering immediate comfort but would never dispose of the same long-term performance as with RGPL. Gigantopapillary conjunctivitis is found in both brands (SCL, RGPL), intolerance has been especially observed with SCL (long-term complication).

Dry eye, frequent at presbyopic age, does not represent a counter-indication towards wearing SCL (prefer low hydrophilia lenses) or RGPL ones or in silicohydrogel SCL.

We can possibly take the time to advise regular artificial tear instillation, preservative-free drops, compatibles with contact lenses; or, under local anesthesia, we can deal with the insertion of lacrymal micro-plugs favoring the natural tears retention, preventing elimination via oculolacrimonasal duct.

Oral hydration and adapted diet, rich in essential polyunsaturated fatty acids (omega-3 and omega-6), found in borage and primrose oils, can also improve local trophic conditions to wear contact lenses.

To reach ideal comfort, presbyope wearing contact lenses must be able to use distant, intermediate and near vision, with his precorneal lenses only.

If not, he would be forced to wear, whether temporarily or permanently, additive spectacles over the contact lenses to compensate optical insufficiency in distant or near vision.

However, this does not look like satisfactory optical solution before having tried different contactological solutions.

There is no standardized solution as far as contact lenses are concerned for presbyopia.

In anisometropias (*See also* paragraph 2.3.3, Maintaining near vision, page 58), we will advise a monovision, that is to say a lens for distant vision on the dominant eye and a lens adapted to near vision on the other eye (*See also* paragraph 3.3.8, Monovision LASIK, page 108).

In other situations, we will prefer to propose bi or multifocal lenses to the presbyopic patient. Multifocal SCLs are based upon different vision principles:

- the most frequent being a central optical zone devoted to near vision (as the accommodation-convergence-miosis synkinesia) and a peripheral zone in distant vision (*See also* paragraph 1.3.1, Synkinesis, page 12),
- the opposite is less frequent (some manufacturers propose a central distant vision in myopes and a peripheral near vision, this type of profile being never applicable to hyperopes),
- or a succession of concentric rings with alternation of the distant and near vision spherical zones for an independent adaptation of the pupillary diameter.

The transition zone between distant vision and near vision can be progressive (powers progressive profile), or abrupt, with variable central multiasphericity.

Additions must take into account values we have found during the examination in aerial optical compensation (*See also* paragraph 3.1, Presbyopia and spectacles, page 80), which we have modified in accordance with a correlation map and the given soft lens.

Same addition profiles are applicable to RGPL, with supplementary possibilities as for the segmented alternate vision (bifocality to right segment on demand).

3.2.4 Orthokeratology (OK) (Fig. 3.4)

Note special mention concerning the nocturnal orthokeratological lenses.

The OK lenses are RGPL, with inverted geometry (more flat in the center than in corneal periphery), many degagement, cell reserves and several concentric zones, enabling a corneal epitheliostromal superficial remodeling.

The OK lenses:

- are worn at night,
- over a duration of at least 5 hours,
- without any discomfort under shut eyelids,
- with centrocorneal flattening effect by a central pressional mechanical effect on the epithelium, leading to a centrifugal migration of cells towards the lens reserve zone.

With nocturnal wearing renewal, in few days, epithelial redistribution, absolutely reversible, comes together with central corneal thinning.

OK lens removal during the day allows these cells to migrate again towards the center with progressive shift in the corrected myopia. This tends to induce a vesperal residual myopia in favor of intermediate and near vision in young presbyopes. Such an optical compensation thus adresses peculiarly low myopes and young presbyopes.

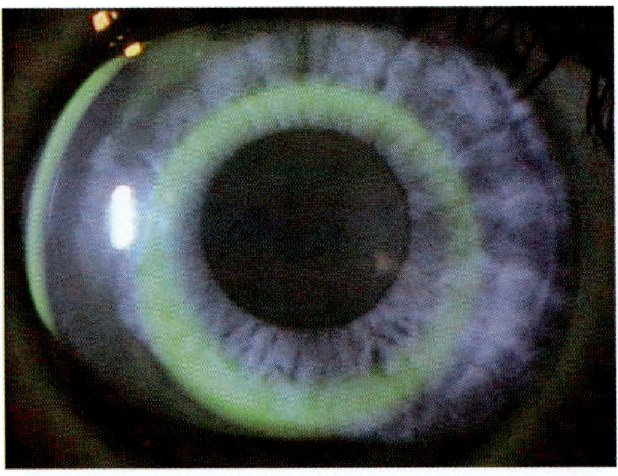

Fig. 3.4 Overnight OK lens on eye examined through biomicroscope with cobalt blue filter after fluorescein instilling (Personal picture obtained on digital RO5000 Rodenstock slit lamp)

OK lens permits night corneal remodeling and effective vision without wearing contact lenses during the day. Central flattening zone enables a myopia optical correction inferior to −4.50 diopters. Annular zone, in fluorescence, corresponds to an area dedicated to collection of epithelial cells after centrifugal migration.

Under the effect of the lenses, the modification of the corneal epithelial diopter controls the loss of power. Besides, nowadays, we perfectly handle this technology.

The OK lenses are recommended:
- for simple myopias inferior to –4.50 diopters,
- with sufficient corneal excentration in the central 30° calculated on anterior videokeratography,
- are available for myopic astigmats as well.

By enabling controlled epithelial remodeling, OK lenses bring to the presbyopic myopes in their forties:
- excellent morning comfort in distant vision (strong morning accommodative capacities),
- good vesperal comfort in near vision (evening accommodative lack).

To accentuate this optical effect, we can facilitate near vision by targeting a residual ametropia permitting a monovision (*See also* paragraph 3.3.2, Monovision, page 95).

Cleaning and hygiene are, the constraints of RGPL but the same as all other type of contact lenses.

We can also propose presbyopia surgery to our patients as alternative to wearing spectacles or contact lenses.

3.3 PRESBYOPIA AND REFRACTIVE SURGERIES

We have to distinguish surgical techniques aimed at this chapter as optical compensation. Accommodation restoration surgical techniques, will be the subject of the following chapter (*See also* paragraph 4.2, Presbyopia and implant accommodative surgeries, page 142).

While waiting for correcting presbyopia, various techniques are here to compensate it, in so far as we choose the right one for the right patient. Although refractive surgery has made considerable progress over the last 15 years, the endless list of techniques proposed shows the absence of consensus.

Some colleagues present presbyopia like a major obstacle to all refractive surgery.

Here are some elements that can contribute to putting this position into question.

First we will classify the different methods of presbyopic compensation refractive surgery according to the target organ, as studied in the previous chapters (*See also* paragraph 1.5.4, Accommodative structures, page 34).

3.3.1 History of Refractive Surgeries

If we briefly remind history, we realize that cornea has triggered many clinical evaluations:
- diamond-knife hexagonal keratotomy (Grady, 1988),
- multifocal refractive photokeratectomy (Moreira, 1992),
- decentered multifocal laser-assisted in situ keratomileusis (LASIK) (Baueberg, 1999),
- conductive keratoplasty (Kommehl, 2004),
- multifocal LASIK with peripheral near vision (Telandro, 2004),
- multifocal LASIK with centered near vision (Alio, 2006).

Crystalline lens has also been an organ studied for presbyopia compensation:
- monovision after cataract surgery (*See* 3.3.2, p. 95),
- Phako-Ersatz (Parel, 1989) (*See also* 4.3.1, p. 153),
- multifocal refractive IOL (Keates, 1987) (*See* 3.3.9.4, p. 114),
- multifocal diffractive IOL (Hansen, 1990),
- lenticular capsuloplasty (Jungschaffer, 1994),
- multifocal phakic IOL (Baïkoff, 2003) (*See* 3.3.9.1, p. 109),
- phakomodulation (Krueger, 2006) (*See also* 4.3.1, p. 153).

By scleral approach the presbyopic surgery techniques, have rather fallen within the competence of accommodative restoration, and we will then study them in the next chapter (*See also* 4.2, p. 142):
- anterior ciliary sclerotomy (Thornton, 1990) (*See also* 4.1.1, p. 138),
- intrascleral siliconed implants (Fukasaku, 1998) (*See also* 4.1.2, p. 139),
- laser assisted sclerotomy (Lim, 1998) (*See also* 4.1.3, p. 140),
- scleral expansion bands (Schachar, 1999) (*See also* 4.2.1, p. 142),
- intrascleral titanium implants (Jory, 2002),
- supraciliary segments (Baïkoff, 2002).

As observed on the chronology above, presbyopic surgery is a relatively recent refractive surgery.

Like all refractive surgery, presbyopia surgery must take into account underlying ametropias and correct them at the same time (*See also* chapter 2, Presbyopia and ametropias, page 44).

3.3.2 Monovision

Monovision consists of favoring the distant vision on the dominant eye and near vision on the other one, especially for the myopes, the anisomyopes, more seldom in hyperopes.

It remains easy to manage it: good vision quality, included in low light.

Disadvantages are secondary to anisometropia induced between both eyes: aniseikonia and fatigability get greater as anisometropia increases.

Anxious subjects, even if good theoretical indications, do not admit a degree of ocular penalization or remove the ambivalent neutralization by frequent spontaneous or voluntary occlusions that disrupt binocular vision.

Next to monovision, there is another presbyopia surgical principle that calls on multifocality, a very fashionable concept at the moment.

3.3.3 Simultaneous Vision

The multifocality is based on the principle of distal, intermediate and proximal simultaneous vision that requires particular cerebral plasticity, and cortical sorting for the cognitive selection of relevant images.

In multifocality, the sharing of focal points can come with:

- the creation of optical zones both concentric and with juxtaposed different powers (refractive optics),
- Fresnel's optical interface that deviates some of the images focal points in secondary point objects (diffractive optics),
- the modulation of higher order optical aberrations such as the negative spherical aberration (optical power superior in the center compared with the periphery to a near vision effect in the center) or the coma (decentering of a spherical aberration contributing to light beams defocusing so that we spread adjacent images focal points) (*See also* paragraph 2.5.6.3, Multifocal WF, page 75).

The multifocality surgically induced constitutes a recent but efficient presbyopia compensation technique on subjects who have been selected beforehand.

Multifocality permits action synergy between both eyes, what tends to provide with a vision more balanced than monovision, a preservation of the distal image on the dominated eye, and better intermediate vision for advanced presbyopes.

However, the loss of contrasts sensitivity is greater in this technique than in monovision due to the light sharing between distal and proximal vision, if a lazy cortical adaptation slows down.

Even though these surgical techniques do not bring strictly speaking presbyopia surgical corrections, it is no less true that surgical compensation is clinically very satisfactory and perfectly meets the refractive goals, expected by patients.

3.3.4 Informed Consent

It is necessary to provide the patients, who are to undergo surgery, with appropriate information. This requires a visual function evaluation beyond the simple keratometrical and a visual acuity test:
- residual and appearing accommodation amplitude,
- eye multifocality and optical quality,
- performance in intermediate vision,
- contrast perception to 10%, 20% and 100% saturation,
- resistance to dazzle.

Multifocality must appear like an optical tip that is about creating irregularities, themselves putting a variety of optics at our disposal for all vision distance.

Whether we classify the surgical methods according to:
- action mode (additive, subtractive, relaxing, contracting),
- action site (cornea, anterior chamber, sclera),
- or action mechanism (monovision, multifocality).

All refractive surgeries are potentially applicable to presbyopia compensation.

Pre- or postoperative functional evaluation is a key point in presbyopia surgery.

A survey about the expectations (possibility to wear occasional complementary correction) and the subjective visual performance (daily tasks with or without spectacles or contact lenses, seeing halos, glare or ghosting, trouble in mesoscotopic condition, visual fatigability) represents invaluable help to assess the patients results and realistic aspect of their expectations.

3.3.5 Preoperative Evaluation

In case of postoperative multifocality, we need to study thoroughly refraction, for the subject has a wide tolerance to different spherocylindrical compensations (defocusing curve, aberrometry) (*See also* paragraph 2.5.6.1, Aberrometry, page 69).

We will also estimate:

- Maximum reading speed, under standardized light, taking into account linguistic adaptations and cognitive abilities (*See also* paragraph 1.4.3.1, Search for maximal accommodation, page 21),
- Contrast sensitivity to 10%, 20% and 100% with visual abilities test (VAT) (*See also* paragraph 1.4.2, Ergonomics, page 20),
- Accommodation amplitude by push-up test or defocusing curve (*See* paragraph 3.1.1, Addition determining, page 80),
- Binocular vision study. Stereoscopic vision is all the more troubled in monovision since anisometropia is strong (do not exceed 2 diopters of induced anisometropia); we must evaluate it in both distant vision and near vision. We have to assess the oculomotor balance near and far, with and without correction, in order to detect dysphorias/tropias, essentially induced in monovision situations.

Tropia, or strabismus, is a permanent or intermittent deviation, while binocular vision is not divided.
Reminder: a dysphoria is a latent deviation (*See* paragraph 3.1.3, Multifocal lenses, page 84).

Sensorial balance of patient is up for presbyopia compensation with monovision by respecting the ocular dominance.

We can figure this predominance thanks to the cylinder test or using the preferential gaze technique: with a –0.75 diopter lens in near vision and +0.75 diopter in distant vision. Eye that is the most troubled in tested vision would not be penalized.

Then, in preoperative time, we will propose candidate a presurgical functional simulation. Contact lenses trial will simulate refractive surgery, respecting the underlying ametropia and in accordance with the technique used (multifocal lenses or monovision with contact lenses trial).

It is essential to take surgical decision with a videokeratoscopia analyzing anterior segment (Pentacam HR, Orbscan), more than a simple corneal topography:

- central keratometries, corneal anterior and posterior faces peripheral keratometries,
- pachymetry mapping all over cornea,
- camerular depth and iridocorneal angle analysis,
- iris structure,
- phakodensitometry (Fig. 3.5),
- corneal aberrometry (*See* Fig. 2.8), and
- mesopic pupillometry (*See also* paragraph 1.3.2, Miosis, page 26).

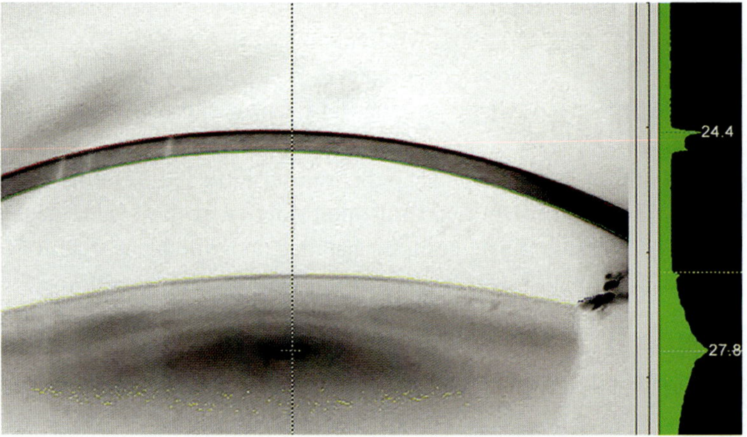

Fig. 3.5 Scheimpflug picture of the anterior segment with phakodensitometrical study (Personal picture obtained with HR Pentacam)

Thanks to this picture of the anterior segment taken according to Scheimpflug technique, we isolate more easily crystalline lens located at the back of the cornea and of the anterior chamber (optically empty space).

A curve (green curve on the right hand of the image) represents the densitometry of the transparent crossed structures.

The opacification peaks of the curve represent the measurement of the crystalline opalescences density (phakodensitometry) along the light path (vertical dotted line).

In this example, central nuclear cataract contributes up to more than 20% of the opacity.

Phakodensitometry: by analogy with bone mineral density test (osteodensitometry), this is the measuring of crystalline lens optical density. We evaluate it with progressive attenuation of the light beam. Step by step, while it crosses eye transparent structures, this beam is incident. Densitometry is expressed in percentage of light attenuation:

- down to 0%, structures are perfectly transparent,
- around 100%, crystalline lens opacity is major (Fig. 3.5).

Corneal biomechanical structure is evaluated with the ocular response analyzer (ORA) (Fig. 3.6), which provides us intrinsic viscoelastical properties of the cornea to operate on: corneal hysteresia showing the corneal ability to get its initial shape back (*See also* 1.5.5, Pseudo-accommodation, page 37).

After air jet induced deformation (between 10 and 12 units), corneal resistance factor is calculated, intraocular pressure (IOP) is estimated from the flattening values (a soft and thin cornea underevaluates intraocular pressure, a thick cornea overevaluates IOP).

We thus determine corneas with unfavorable biomechanical profile to any keratosurgery: minimal keratopachymetry compromises postoperative architectonic stability regarding the photoablation that is proportional to the ametropia to treat. Moreover, the ablation is completed for presbyopia treatment (additive corneal laser treatment).

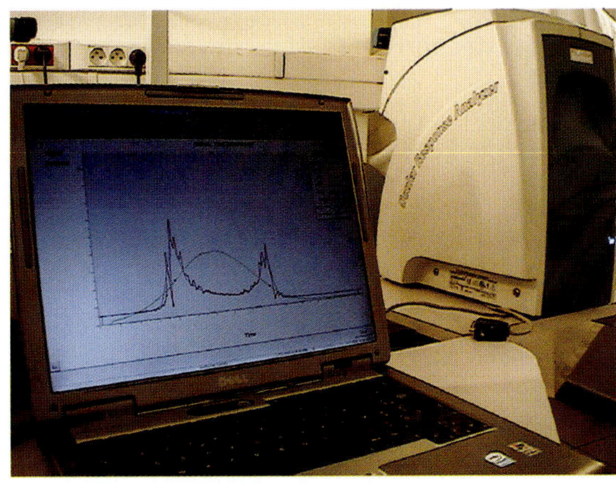

Fig. 3.6 Device for ocular response analysis (ORA) as examination prior to refractive surgery (Personal picture of the ORA commercialized by Reichert and sold by EBC company in France)

Today, ORA is the only device up to now that allows to estimate corneal biomechanical characteristics. Based on the reflectometrical response after pneumatic stimulus (green "bell" curve on the screen). Cornea depresses and inverts its curvature before taking back its initial position. It then goes on with two plane states corresponding to the two red peaks.

After reasoned argumentation, not ideal cases for laser refractive surgery, can then go for different technique that does not concern cornea (phake implantation for instance) (*See* paragraph 3.3.9, Lenticular surgeries, page 109).

3.3.6 Keratosurgical Lasers

Let us now approach presbyopia surgery via *excimer* laser subtractive corneal treatment.

Laser corneal surgery principle is well established: corneal tissue irreversible and controlled ablation, by *excited dimer* (excimer) laser disruption emitting a 193-nm radiation invisible wave.

After correcting myopia with laser treatment, cornea, naturally aspherical and oblate (center more curved than periphery), tends to become prolate (periphery more curved than central cornea) and less aspherical (*See also* paragraph 2.5.6.2, Spherical aberrations, page 73).

Asphericity is a geometrical model that opposes sphericity. We call spherical all geometrical shape fitting in a sphere with a given radius. We call aspherical all geometrical shape that fits in several spheres with given radii. If the curvature radii are more and more arched from the center to the periphery, the asphericity is prolate, the opposite being oblate.

Peripheral tissue subtraction that stems from hyperopic laser correction emphasizes the corneal central curvature.

Since the eighties, when the first trials of excimer laser keratorefractive treatments took place, many technological improvements have contributed to optimize (Fig. 3.7):
- photodisruption quality (energy, fluence),
- the speed of laser optic oscillations and their accuracy (active *eye-tracker*), the stability of laser generative cavities (gaseous mix, *solid state*),
- the improvement of the ablative profits and overriding control (Gaussian spots, customized treatments).

However, tissular target still remains today a controversial subject: which corneal structure (epithelium, Bowman's membrane, anterior stroma, posterior stroma) to ablate?

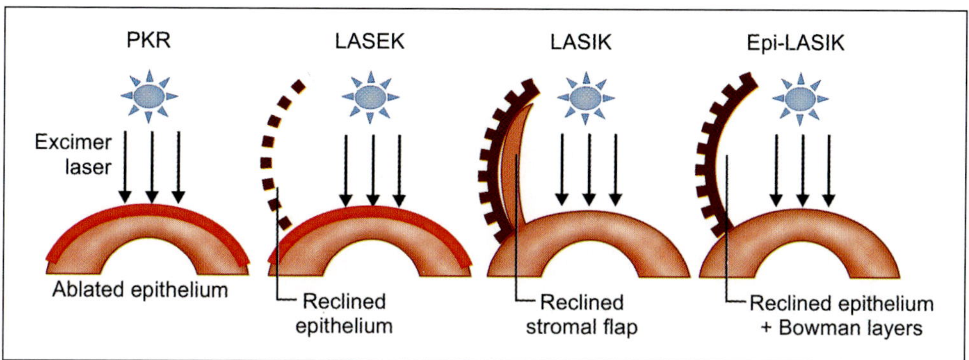

Fig. 3.7 Schematical principles of four excimer laser keratorefractive surgeries

Corneal surface supporters (refractive photokeratectomy or RPK, *Laser assisted epithelial keratomileusis* or LASEK, *epithelial laser assisted in situ keratomileusis* or epi-LASIK) give:

- more security,
- enhancement procedure,
- a slight risk of ectatic complication despite more frequent haze.

For the others (*Laser assisted intrastromal keratomileusis* or LASIK, femtosecond assisted LASIK or femtoLASIK), intrastromal treatment, with a depth that is better and better controlled, remains the gold standard in refractive keratosurgery.

LASIK remains the reference as far as refractive surgery is concerned in the United States and in Europe, bosting a lot of operations each year.

The popularity of this procedure arises from advantages:

- painless process (then often bilateral intervention),
- quick visual rehabilitation (just a few hours with LASIK compared with days or weeks with surface technique).

LASIK was initially inspired by the Hispanic ophthalmologist Joaquim Barraquer's intrastromal surgeries (keratomileusis). The Cretan ophthalmologist Ioannis Pallikaris invented LASIK back in the eighties.

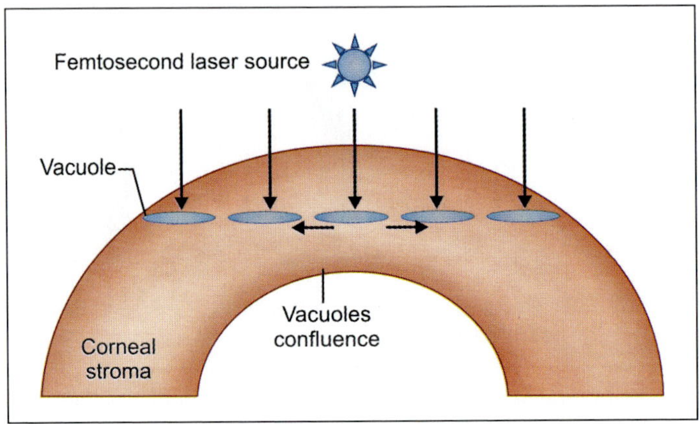

Fig. 3.8 Femtosecond laser's principle of tissular cutting on the cornea

The cutting of a corneal flap, in thickness controlled (Fig. 3.8) (110 μm respecting a posterior stromal wall after ablation thicker than 250 μm), and the linking hinge (to avoid all suture) that lies in the nasal or corneal superior area, can unfold with the help of:

- a steel blade (microkeratome),
- high pressure water jet or,
- ultra rapid laser (Femtosecond 'FS' laser).

The notion of residual posterior wall after corneal laser surgery is a condition to be respected in order to avoid long-term corneal ectasia.

Stromal interface quality, accuracy and security of the corneal flap cut favor FS laser. Indeed, after centering the laser apparatus head on the cornea and temporary support suction, it can carry out an intrastromal interface by confluent vacuolization in 15 seconds.

FS laser is an ultrafast pulsed laser (10–15 sec) that enables an accurate cutting of the corneal stromal tissue by vaporization without heating.

Technological advance as far as femtoLASIK is concerned (LASIK with prior FS laser cut of the flap) should allow to envisage, not only a tissular ablation, but also a stromal lenticule ablation, which would permit a real intraLASIK (REmoval Lens EXchange).

Once ametropia corrected with one of these techniques in distant vision, presbyopia may or may not benefit from a multifocal presbyLASIK for near vision.

3.3.7 PresbyLASIK (Figs 3.9A and B)

The optical principle of corneal surgical compensation lies in the control of the beam lights division:
- induction of a myopia on the dominated eye (monovision responsible for a biocular pseudo-accommodation) (*See* paragraph 3.3.8, Monovision LASIK, page 108),
- induction of a negative spherical aberration and of a coma on each eye (multifocality responsible for monocular pseudo-accommodation) (*See also* paragraph 2.5.6.3, Multifocal WF, page 75).

Pseudo-accommodation (*See also* paragraph 1.5.5, page 37) is an optical mechanism that may require the intervention of both eyes (biocular pseudo-accommodation), or each eye separately (monocular pseudo-accommodation).

These two methods can combine with the multifocality on the dominated eye and the emmetropia on the dominant one, what offers several advantages in terms of lesser binocularity impairment:
- better distal vision with low contrast on dominant eye,
- better intermediate vision under low contrast.

Multifocal presbyLASIK concerns in priority emmetrope or low hyperope, monovision LASIK involves mainly myopes.

With multifocal presbyLASIK, several ablative profiles are optional for hyperopic presbyope or hyperopic astigmat, emmetrope, myope or myopic astigmat.

I personally use a mix of different ablative profiles according to:
- the extent of the underlying ametropia (*See also* chapter 2, p. 44),
- actual pre-existing anisometropia (*See also* 2.3.3, p. 58),

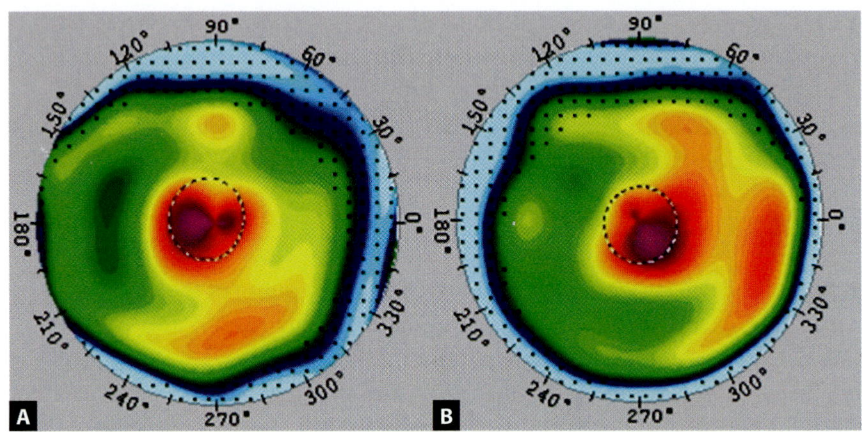

Figs 3.9A and B PresbyLASIK off-centered and centered topographical hyperopic examples (Personal maps obtained with a subtraction of the digital topographical images from the Pentacam driver software)

Elevation differential topographies, orangey color shows the hypermetropical ablation zone in distant vision, dotted central circle defines pupillary area, and purple color illustrates off-centered ablation zone as inferior nasal on topography A, centered ablation zone on pupillary area for near vision (topography B).

Being the same patient, the dominant right eye A rapidly recovers a satisfactory distant vision because, without miosis, distal vision is clear whereas, in postoperative time, the left eye B got back greater near vision acuity and delayed penalization in distant vision.

- anterior segment analysis data (*See* 3.3.5, p. 97),
- mesopic pupillometry (*See also* 1.3.2, p. 13).

In low hyperopes and presbyopic emmetropes, we may propose ablative profile with addition for off-centered near vision on dominant eye, ablative profile with addition for centered near vision on dominant eye, ablative profile for centered near vision on the dominated eye.

On the dominant eye, in the nasal inferior zone of pupil, the addition surface is shifted around 1 mm. This is a theoretical advantage, for not only does it follow the pupillary moving during the accommodation convergence-miosis synkinesis (*See also* paragraph 1.3.1, Synkinesis, page 12), but also it frees the visual axis in distal vision.

On the dominated eye, we possibly administer correction for hyperopia over a wide area (until 9.5 mm when the anatomical conditions allow it) centered for distant vision.

Consecutively, concentrically to distant treatment, we provide surgically a centered addition. This treatment impairs distant vision for a rather long time.

In myopes, the most reluctant patients to near vision loss, and after trial of contact lenses correcting presbyopia in central or peripheral near vision, we may propose:

- whether an ablative profile by subtraction with centered distant vision in which centered hyperopic treatment follows overcorrective myopic treatment (peripheral distant vision, central near vision),
- or hyperopic treatment following an undercorrective myopic one (peripheral near vision, centered distant vision).

In delicate and difficult cases, the simulation with contact lenses test allows to choose the least penalizing treatment in accordance with the patients expectation.

Laser devices to use are just important in the treatment procedure (surgeon dependant).

The effect of the ablative profile are checked on the cornea with videokeratotopography by means of elevation maps (Figs 3.9A and B).

In the centered presbyLASIK, addition surface is centered on the pupil in distant vision, but decentered in near during miosis.

In the decentered presbyLASIK, addition surface is centered on the pupil in accommodative miosis, but the pupil remains free in distant vision.

The aforementioned ablative profiles induce the formation of defocusing optical higher order aberrations (positive and negative spherical aberrations, coma) that are beneficial to near vision, but require adaptation delay for distant vision.

In presbyopes operated on for myopic LASIK, we obtain the multifocality to the detriment of the proximal vision (oblate cornea, positive spherical aberration), while in presbyopes operated on for hyperopic LASIK, induced multifocality favors a contrario field depth and proximal vision (hyper-prolate cornea, negative spherical aberration) (*See also* paragraph 2.5.6.2, Spherical aberrations, page 73).

Presbyopes operated on for presbyLASIK thus must be able to benefit for aberrometrical measures in perioperative time according to the pupillary diameter.

Presbyopic emmetropes operated on for presbyLASIK, show a preoperative positive spherical aberration correction on aberrometry.

The induced negative spherical aberration due to multifocal presbyLASIK presbyopic emmetropes generates:

- a myopic pupil in near vision (miosis) and (*See also* paragraph 1.3.2, Miosis, page 13),
- an emmetropic pupillary periphery in distal vision (relative mydriasis),
- the intermediate vision in the transitional zone between the two previous.

Within the scope of an out-centered presbyLASIK, the iatrogenic induction of an inferior nasal oblique coma corresponds topographically to bifocal cornea, in favor of near vision (*See also* paragraph 2.5.6.1, Aberrometry, page 69).

To create a multifocality necessary to presbyopic compensation, presbyLASIK must come with hyper-prolate corneal surface: more arched in the center than normal cornea treated with monofocal hyperopic LASIK: great asphericity, from –0.80 to 1.00 (normal corneal asphericity coefficient being Q = –0.13).

Optical results depend on the operative technique:

- monofocal hyperopic LASIK improves near vision thanks to the induction of negative spherical aberration (prolate cornea),
- decentered presbyLASIK gets an excellent near visual acuity, to the detriment of distant vision, at least during the first three postoperative months,
- up to 10% contrast, distant vision gets back to normal after 2 years with a monofocal hyperopic LASIK, while, for multifocal presbyLASIKs, it remains inferior to 1 or 2 lines on the logMAR scale (*See also* paragraph 1.4.1, Measures, page 19),
- reading speed is normal in all hyperopic presbyopic patients or emmetropes operated on for centered or decentered presbyLASIK, with accommodation amplitude increased and improvement of the refractive defocusing curve.

This is why we advise presbyLASIK to low hyperopes (inferior to +3.50 diopters) or to emmetropes:

- if more than 50 and less than 65 years old (starting cataract age),
- if moderate astigmatism (inferior to +2.50),
- if better visual acuity between 20/20 with 90% contrast and, as a minimum, 2/10 and 10% contrast,
- if no contraindication for excimer laser treatments on cornea, no keratectasia, or flat/curved cornea (power between 39 and 46 diopters),

- if no systemic disease affecting collagen or chronic inflammatory disease, and/or current treatment with medication interfering with wound healing process (corticoids, antimitotics, non-steroidal anti-inflammatory drugs, pregnancy).

If, for myopic presbyope, we opt for an excimer laser solution: propose monovision LASIK.

In case of starting or manifest cataract, crystalline lens extraction with implantation of a multifocal new brand IOL is a longer lasting solution.

Crystalline lens extraction technique may occur after a presbyLASIK, but should make us double check the choice parameters of IOL with special nomogram (Haigis parameters on IOL master for instance). We will come back to it later (Fig. 3.17).

In the situation of postoperative result not meeting the patient expectations, and after resuming presbyLASIK by aberrometry-guided photoablation, it is always possible to proceed with an ablative treatment neutralizing the refractive effects.

Keratorefractive laser is a tissular ablation irreversible technique.

Despite potential complications and tissular disorganization that will persist, we can still propose a new laser treatment to erase the effects of the previous treatment.

For presbyopic myope, apart from monovision solution, it is possible to propose centered presbyLASIK treatment including:

- overcorrecting ablative profile of about –1.50 diopters (peripheral near vision with induced hyperopia of +1.50 diopters) over wide optical zone,
- and concentric hypermetropic treatment of 1.50 diopters, over small optical zone (central distant vision).

With this treatment, most of our patients get a good compensation in distant vision, 20% have lost one visual acuity line, 3 patients out of 4 can read Jaeger 3 without correction, with a final asphericity reduced,[5] in case of initial myopia inferior to –5.00 diopters.

Asphericity in the 20° central cornea is equivalent to eccentricity, that is to say a coefficient quantifying the curvature change from the center to the corneal periphery.

Satisfaction survey brings 85% of patients who feel an improvement in vision, 15% complain about night halos.

Despite these considerations presbyLASIK turns out to be an efficient optical compensation for presbyopia. It works by the change of corneal curvature the modulation of the HOA (*See also* paragraph 2.5.6.1, Aberrometry, page 69), to optimize natural multifocality and render distant and near vision without correction.

PresbyLASIK is then particularly interesting for low hyperopes and emmetropes for it represents a theoretically reversible solution, less intrusive than clear lens surgery (multifocal IOL implantation) (*See* paragraph 3.3.9, Lenticular surgeries, page 109).

3.3.8 Monovision LASIK

Monovision LASIK constitutes asymmetrical approach concerning negative spherical aberration (*See also* paragraph 2.5.6.2, Spherical aberrations, page 73) and oblique coma on dominant eye to:
- improve the field depth (*See* paragraph 3.3.9, Lenticular surgeries, page 109) and the near vision without correction,
- preserve a good distal visual acuity, and
- insure a satisfactory binocular contrasts sensitivity.

Some authors develop new ablative techniques with excimer laser that could be a good solution for presbyopes.

The induction of a positive spherical aberration (*See also* paragraph 2.5.6.1, Aberrometry, page 69) could compensate accommodative loss in presbyopia without exceeding the addition of 2.00 diopters.

With this technique, it seems easier to correct myopic eyes than hyperopic. Moreover, usual excimer laser myopic correction increases negative spherical aberration.

The handling of spherical aberration, to induce it more positive, simultaneously reduces the increase in negative spherical aberration. Consequently, resulting cornea will be more prolate than expected with a pure myopic correction, then mimicking physiological corneal curvature.

If, for now (*See also* 2.5.6.3, Multifocal WF, page 75), adaptative optics sticks to clinical research, its wide application field lets us foresee numerous possibilities for diagnosis and therapies in visual optics.

Some authors have had presbyopic compensation method patented. Technique comes down to inducing a controlled rate of HOA at the level of the ocular wavefront (*See also* paragraph 2.5.6.3, Multifocal WF, page 75).

In this method, adaptative optics gives possibility to test a patient about different motives and multifocal corrective powers before any definitive making of a lens, of an IOL or of a customized multifocal photoablative treatment.

Beside excimer laser presbyopic surgery, there are other surgical techniques interesting cornea, whether directly (IOLs implants in pseudophakes) or indirectly phakic IOLs in phakes (from the Greek: the crystalline lens), concerning the crystalline lens. All are qualified as intraocular lenses (IOLs).

3.3.9 Lenticular Surgeries

We surgically position phakic IOLs in front of the crystalline lens left intact.

We insert pseudophake IOLs in place of the natural crystalline lens. This lens will also play the part of artificial crystalline lens (IOL).

After crystalline lens ablation and in the lack of IOL, we qualify the subject as aphakic.

Today, presbyopic lenticular techniques use three implants entities (Fig. 3.10):

- phakic implants are to be inserted between crystalline lens and cornea (phakic IOLs),
- monopseudophakic implant is to be placed instead of extracted crystalline lens (IOL), and
- bipseudophakic implant is to be standing before an IOL already in place (IOL *piggy-back*).

3.3.9.1 Phakic IOLs

Monopseudophakia: eye implanted with a single IOL.

Bipseudophakia: eye implanted with a pair of IOLs:

- two IOLs in capsular bag or,
- one IOL in capsular bag and one lens in the ciliary sulcus (*See also* Fig. 4.25, page 163).

There are several distinct types of IOLs called phakic because associated with a clear crystalline lens in place, and according to the site of implantation:

- posterior chamber phakic IOL (space between iris posterior surface and crystalline lens anterior surface, which the ciliary sulcus borders outside) is placed between the anterior crystalloid and the posterior iris pigment epithelium (Fig. 3.11),

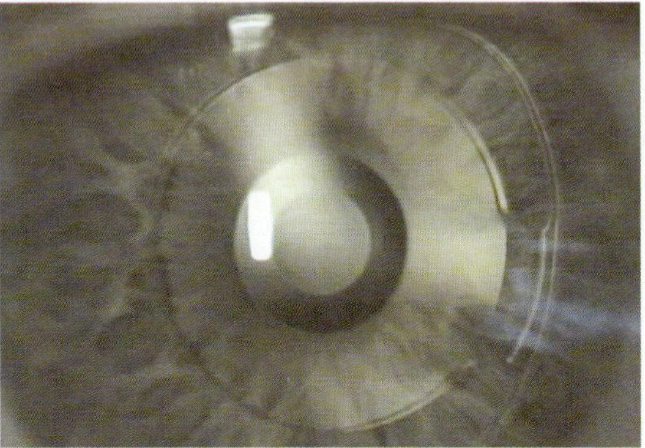

Fig. 3.10 Multifocal anterior chamber phakic IOL (personal iconography taken from a Rodenstock 5000 slit lamp mounted with a CCD camera)

This anterior chamber bifocal phakic IOL has been microsurgically placed between cornea and iris plane. Optic is perfectly centered at the very middle of the pupil, haptics maintain the intraocular device with synthetic material micropodes lying in the iridocorneal angle. This type has proven its efficacy in compensating presbyopia in low ametropias but is no longer implanted due to long-term side effects.

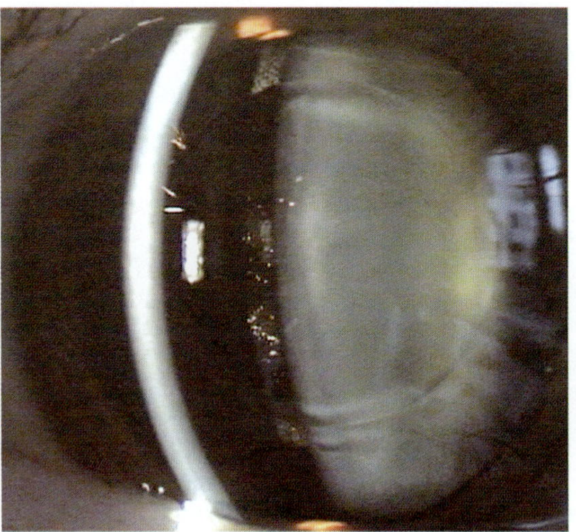

Fig. 3.11 Phakic refractive lens (PRL) IOL in place observed behind a large dilated pupil (personal iconography taken from a Rodenstock 5000 slit lamp mounted with a CCD camera)

This posterior chamber monofocal phakic IOL has been microsurgically placed between the crystalline lens and the iris plane. Melanin pigments deposits are clearly seen on the anterior surface of the optic, haptics take place in the ciliary sulcus. This type has not been developed for presbyopic compensation.

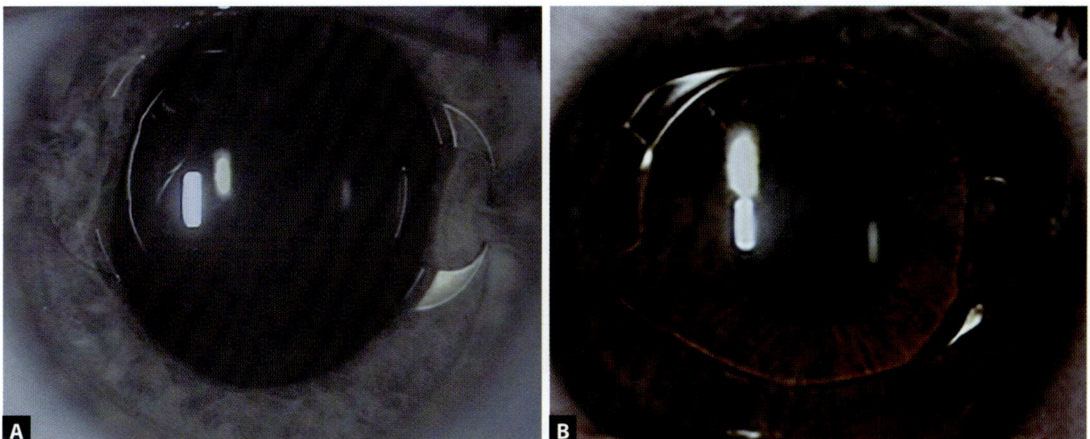

Figs 3.12A and B Iris-claw Phakic IOL in place on a dilated (A) and non-dilated pupil (B)
(Personal iconography taken from a Rodenstock 5000 slit lamp mounted with a CCD camera)

This iris-claw monofocal phakic IOL has been microsurgically placed between cornea and pupil. Pharmacological pupil dilation remains effective for fundus oculi examination. Although its safety, this type of IOL has not been developed for presbyopic compensation yet.

- iris phakic IOL is fixed to iris by haptic enclavement as an iris claw (Figs 3.12A and B),
- anterior chamber phakic IOL is positioned ahead of iris with fixations in the camerular angle (Fig. 3.10).

The different types of phakic IOLs are useful to compensate presbyopia in monovision, however, only the anterior chamber phakic IOL used multifocal technology to improve presbyopic visual comfort (Fig. 3.10).

Although these IOLs have had excellent functional results with a patient satisfactory rate superior to 90% (scarcely reached with the present keratorefractive surgery techniques), ANSM (National Agency for Drug and Health products Security) were informed about a corneal endothelium cellular loss in presbyopic patients who had undergone a surgery with these anterior chamber phakic multifocal IOLs.

This organization has then called on all the manufacturers to establish a semestrial follow-up of implanted patients in France and abroad between january 1st, 2003 and december 31st, 2005 (myopia and hyperopia), in order to quantify the endothelial loss frequency and identify the cause.

With these IOLs, some clinical worsening situations have appeared:

- pupil ovalization,
- goniosynechias,
- minimal inflammation with progressive endothelial losses,
- or, on the contrary, a sharp drop in cellular count, after a satisfactory and refractive stability period.

From the optical point of view, this multifocal IOL gave excellent vision, with unchanged accommodation enabling the optimization of the refractive result while keeping outstanding field depth.

Field depth: clearness on both sides of an item.

In early presbyopia, the respect of a security distance between the posterior side of the IOL and the anterior part of the crystalline lens (security zone) could play a decisive role in selecting patients at risk for surgery. The risk is in relation with crystalline lens swelling with age (narrow anterior chamber in hyperopic presbyope and iridocorneal angle closure).

With more rigorous selection criteria of patients the development of phakic multifocal IOLs should regain popularity.

Nevertheless, the removal of these phakic IOLs from the market has not put into question the efficiency and good tolerance of the other implantable devices, even if, in France, they suffer from a great distrust as toward the ophthalmologists as of the patients themselves.

In patients with high hyperopia or myopia implanted with phakic IOLs, the refractive efficiency and the excellent visual quality of the postoperative vision is well known and need no further proof.

3.3.9.2 Mastering Corneal Astigmatism

While operating myopia or hyperopia, astigmatism may be reduced by a corneal approach (single or multiple limbal relaxing incision on the most curved corneal hemi meridian axis) (Fig. 3.13) .

Indeed, such a corneal incision parallel to the limbus induces a flattening in the axis of the corresponding hemimeridian.

The satisfactory control of the corneal approach for IOL introduction enables the concomitant adjustment of preoperative astigmatism.

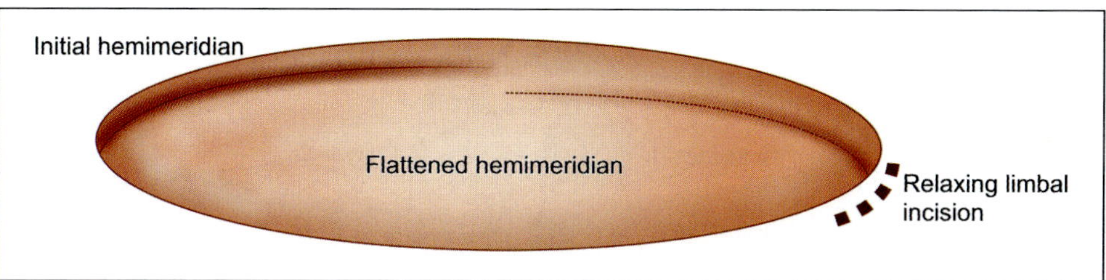

Fig. 3.13 Relaxing limbal incision (large leaders) and its corneal flattening effect (hemimeridian in fine leaders)

According to our experience, a small limbal incision of 3.5 to 4 mm permits a surgical correction of 0.75 to 1.25 diopter corneal astigmatism, a 6-millimeter aperture leads to a surgical correction of 1.75 to 2.00 diopter corneal astigmatism and to 3.00 diopters in case of diametrically opposed limbal incision.

If anti-astigmatism technique has an obvious efficiency, it is all but accurate. This is why other corneal incision techniques but not penetrating were used, to compensate astigmatisms:

- straight transverse keratotomy,
- or arc-shaped incisions (arcuatome, femtolaser).

3.3.9.3 IOLs Piggy-backing

Besides phakic IOLs, the introduction of *piggy-back* multifocal IOLs, in 1997, opened up new horizons to pseudo-accommodative bipseudophakia (*See also* 1.5.5, Pseudo-accommodation, p. 37).

Piggy-backing is a neologism evoking the overlapped implantation of two IOLs to carry out a bipseudophakia.

Bipseudophakic pseudo-accommodation would be connected to the multifocality induced by four optical interfaces, even if the two IOLs are monofocal by themselves (Fig. 3.14).

Initially in rigid and large size PMMA, IOLs were then generating high post-astigmatism (wide corneal incision) unfavorable for presbyopia compensation.

Since then, we have successfully inserted new multifocal soft and foldable IOLs:

- in the capsular bag (during crystalline lens surgery with a double implant insertion, and the materials of which are close/identical for biocompatibility reason),

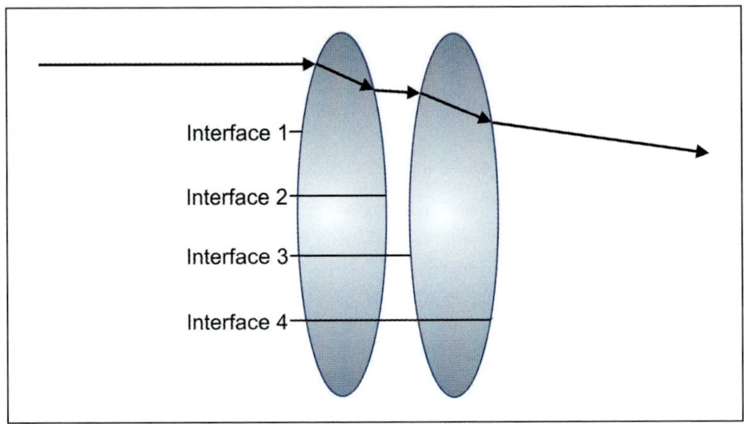

Fig. 3.14 Bipseudophakia benefitting from pseudo-accommodative properties

- or in the ciliary sulcus after or concomitant to crystalline lens surgery (with soft or hard IOL already set in the capsular bag).

Differed indications above all arise from the patients need and their motivation to get a vision without spectacles, on the occasion of first surgery or enhancement.

If zonule is intact and post-surgical residual astigmatism under control, a certain pseudo-accommodation degree appears in bipseudophake (Fig. 3.14), although it causes a decrease in vision quality.

Thanks to our experience, the main complication, albeit exceptional, consits of constitution of interlenticular membrane, compromising the sight, even if the compatibility of both biomaterials was respected.

The ablation of such a membrane occurring in the empty space between the two IOLs consists of a membranectomy aided by accurate focusing by Nd:YAG disruptive laser (Fig. 3.15).

3.3.9.4 Multifocal IOLs

Pseudophakic multifocal IOLs are indicated in:

- spherical ametropias (low astigmatism inferior to 1 diopter) of the presbyope between 50 and 65 years old (beyond, cerebral adaptation is unsure),

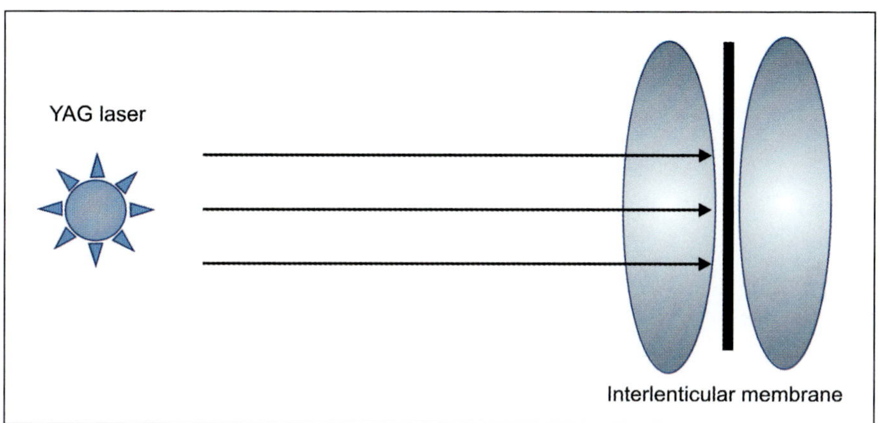

Fig. 3.15 YAG Laser destructive principle of an interlenticular membrane

- high hyperopia or myopia, and
- together with a certain degree of crystalline lens opacification [convincing and medicolegal interest in Scheimpflug phakodensitometry in pictures (*See* Fig. 3.5, page 98)].

Amongst these indications, astigmatisms higher than 1 diopter will need additive surgery, if neglected far vision would turn out to be imperfect in this type of phako-refractive surgery.

Pseudophakic multifocal IOLs correspond to the optically multifocal artificial crystalline lenses. The principle of phako-refractive surgery is to replace the natural crystalline lens with IOL giving emmetropia and the minimal visual aid in near vision.

We will disqualify straightaway for surgery all monophtalm patients, pilots, occupations based upon aiming, night jobs, patients with unrealistic expectations, ocular organical pathologies, wide angle phorias and constitutional or acquired mydriasis.

In all these situations, a phako-refractive surgery without incident could prove inadequate to the expected optical comfort.

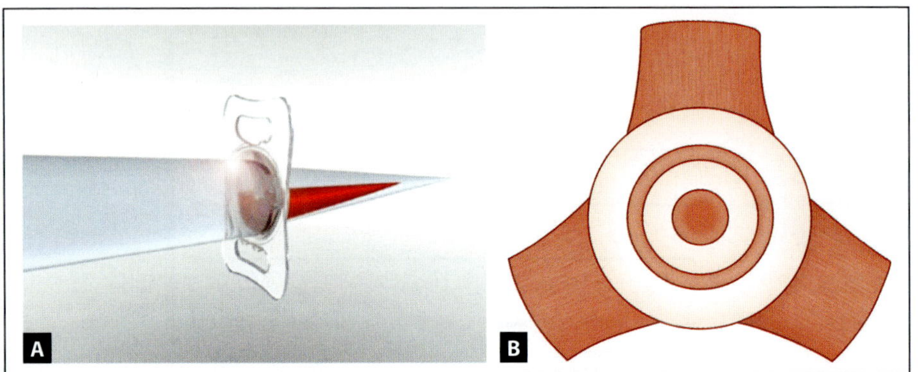

Figs 3.16A and B Examples of bisegmented (Mplus, A) and tripartitioned (MF4, B) multifocal IOLs

Bisegmented IOL (A) must be implanted accurately in the position shown above in order to allow near vision in the inferior part of the device (schematically colored in red). Tripartioned IOL (B) presents concentric zones from center to periphery designed specifically for near, intermediate and far vision.

At present, there are several conceptions of pseudophakic multifocal IOLs:
- refractive implants made up of several concentrical optical zones,
- diffractive implants on Fresnel's physical model, and
- segmented and partitioned implants to express bi or tri focality (Figs 3.16A and B).

The conception of the refractive IOLs works on different curvature radii of the anterior side to determine complementary optical powers for far and near vision, so as to minimize the pupillometric effect over the available quantity of incident light for each zone.

With recent improvements, the diameters of concentric zones have shrunk from the center to the periphery, regarding brand new materials as hydrophilic or hydrophobic acrylic.

The efficiency of the diffractive IOLs is theoretically independent of the pupillary diameter and the dislocation.

Multifocal diffractive optics use a phenomenon based on the undulatory nature of light and lays upon Huygens-Fresnel's physical principle: if light wave-front meets perforated obstacle, one part of light is interrupted, while the rest of it spreads through the system and subdivides itself in several secondary waves of lower amplitude. A diffractive structure interferes to give a new division of light energy.

Diffractive IOLs:
- can combine with refractive zones to increase their optical properties,
- others may own a "natural" yellow filter for a better ultraviolet filtration,
- others propose diffractive apodized steps (reduction of the steps height towards the periphery), balancing the distribution of light energy according to the pupillometry, in order to reduce dysphotopsy and glare, and
- eventually others present a prolate anterior surface to minimize the positive spherical aberration that the crystalline lens extraction induces or propose an optimized aspherical optic to reduce the dysphotopsies, the halos and glares (*See also* paragraph 2.5.6.1, Aberrometry, page 69).

The apodization meets with the fact that diffractive steps height decreases from center to periphery.

This optical characteristic is well known for it reduces the optical aberrations, especially the retina projection of the light rays corresponding to the near vision focal spot, when pupil widens.

As a result, there is a dramatic improvement of night side effects.

Besides, main studies relate 85% of patients autonomy as much for distant vision as near one.

Bad reputation that we generally associate to multifocal IOLs is essentially related to night side effects such as halos or glares.

When pupil is dilated, side effects come along with the undesirable focal spot light rays projected on the retina for near vision, whereas the patient looks in the distance.

Recent technological innovations give the multifocal IOLs a revival of interest.

Regarding the necessary investments this type of technology implies to develop, we can say premium IOLs additional cost is justified, although their partial reimbursement probably also slows down their diffusion.

Hydrophilic or hydrophobic acrylic IOLs are injectable by microincision as wide as between 1.8 and 2.8 mm, after being folded in cartridge designed for this purpose.

The small size of the corneal incision has many advantages:
- quick visual rehabilitation because of low induced astigmatism and
- small corneal wound healing improving resistance and solidity.

Phakosurgery with corneal micro- or mini-incision has enabled the phakorefractive surgery to emarge. Small corneal incisions has rendered necessary to modernize surgical act (bimanual, microcoaxial surgery) and soft IOL implantation to be developed.

3.3.9.5 Surgical Pearls with IOL

Successful and efficient multifocal IOLs lay on the controlled limit of the light dispersion in focal spots (distant, intermediate and near).

Multifocal IOLs must respect:
- perfectly drawn and worked out geometry (*See also* Fig. 4.12),
- echographic biometric implant calculation (mode A unidirectional echography, mode B bidirectional one) (*See also* paragraph 1.5.3, Clinical approach, page 32) or laser (laser interferometry) (Fig. 3.17),
- perfect mastery of postoperative residual astigmatism as seen before (*See* paragraph 3.3.9, Lenticular surgeries, page 109), and
- long-term clear posterior capsule (*See also* paragraph 1.5.1, History, page 28).

Individual expectations enable us to optimize optical compromise:
- motivation to free from optical compensation systems (spectacles, contact lenses),
- understanding of the multifocality principle (as opposed to monofocality),
- realistic functional expectations, and
- neurosensorial and cognitive performance for a satisfactory visual management.

Some reckon we obtain a better multifocality by combining the refractive/diffractive principles on each side: *mix and match.*

Even more than for cataract surgery, the perfect balance of the IOL power is of paramount importance to obtain the expected refractive effect, especially for multifocal IOLs.

Precision does not come without exact preoperative measurements conditioning postoperative emmetropia and pseudo-accommodation effect.

The choice of the calculation formulas for multifocal IOLs is fundamental but is not much distinct from the mathematical formulas we use in IOLs forecast power.

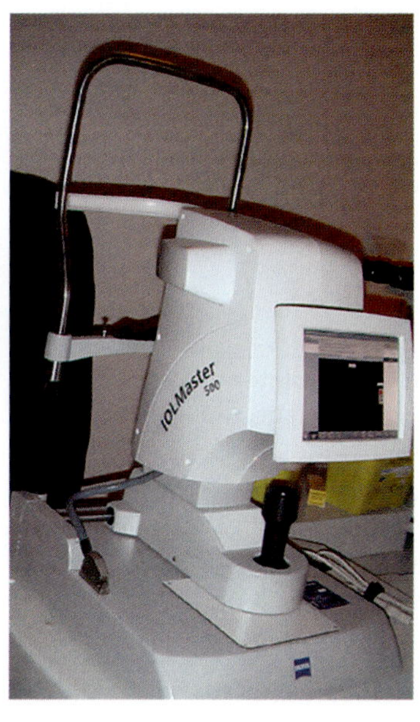

Fig. 3.17 IOL master device for accurate measurement of IOL power to be calculated for emmetropia (Personal iconography taken in the office)

Since echobiometers, IOL master is the only optoelectronic device which provide high accuracy in ocular measurement (keratometry, axial length, anterior chamber depth, lens thickness, white to white diameter) to calculate IOL power for optimal results.

In the past, SRKT formula was used exclusively for myopes, SRK II for emmetropes, the Hoffer Q formula for hyperopes.

In the present, Holladay Haigis-L formula takes into account overall post-keratorefractive modifications.

Some advise surgeons to determine their own calculation constant ("personal constant") in order to customize IOL adaptation, others prefer to average the existing formulas to get as close as possible to refractive aim.

Diffractive IOL centering is absolutely imperative: continuous circular capsulorhexis (cutting of the crystalline lens anterior capsule) must be perfectly centered and of correct size to border the optic (between 5 and 6 mm), in order to ensure correct centering and long-term IOL stability.

Capsulorhexis: surgical technique used to open crystalline lens anterior capsule after carrying out an incision. Quite ordinarily, we regularly rip this capsule with micro-forceps or a needle following a continuous curvilinear path (Fig. 3.18).

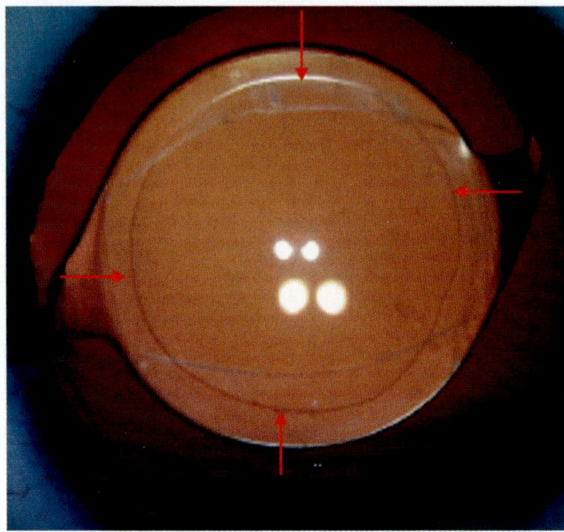

Fig. 3.18 Visible aperture of the anterior capsule of the crystalline lens drawing a roundshape capsulorrhexis (red arrows) in front of IOL

Adequate hand-made capsulorrhexis is necessary for good centration of the IOL and stability with time. Laser capsulorrhexis has been developed to obtain reproducibility and perfect circular capsulorrhexis.

The thorough polishing of the anterior and posterior capsules in the crystalline lens bag with the handpiece or the canula would (Fig. 3.19):

- avoid all capsular contraction (capsulophimosis),
- prevent IOL dislocation due to capsular contraction, and
- delay the posterior capsular opacification (PCO), cause of visual impairment.

Despite all the innovations in matter of IOL surgery the progressive constitution of a secondary cataract (posterior capsular opacification) remains a challenge.

This biological phenomenon generates intensive research to control all the aspects of PCO.

Added with distilled water rinsing (epithelial osmolysis) and thanks to the effect on epithelial cell migration, in some cases, the insertion of a capsular tension ring in the capsular bag would avoid PCO.

As far as functional rehabilitation is concerned, optical results with multifocal IOLs are most satisfactory. Some IOLs are more efficient in distant vision, others in near vision, other again in intermediate vision justifying a combination to cover all the field depth desired.

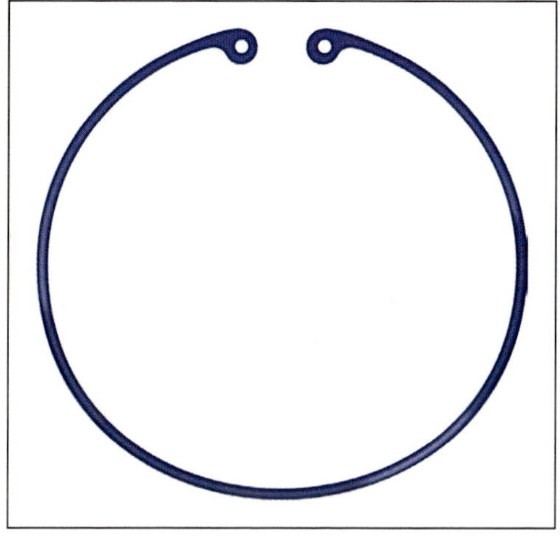

Fig. 3.19 Blue PMMA capsular tension ring prior to implantation in the eye

The insertion in the capsular bag of a capsular tension ring allows an optimal centration of the IOL, delaying PCO and preventing phimosis.

Each IOL shows specific defocusing curve. Compared with other refractive surgeries, multifocal IOLs gain the following advantages:

- ease of implementation (relatively basic surgery for experienced practitioners),
- fast visual rehabilitation,
- efficient vision acuity and quality without correction (especially in case of associated cataract, excellent vision quality for hyperopias higher than +3.00 diopters),
- long-term refractive stability, and
- reimbursement in case of duly certificated cataract.

Multifocal IOLs however have disadvantages:

- more invasive surgery than surface laser surgeries,
- risk of endophthalmitis (endocular infection) statistically estimated at 2‰ (less since intracamerular cefuroxime injection),
- low risk of retinal detachment or edema,
- other eye to be operated in a short delay within a minimum of a week (all the more since the high ametropia or anisometropia is far from supported),

- residual accommodation loss (before 50 years old), and
- more expansive (in 2013 in France the price for a premium IOL varies from 200 to 600 €/US), not including the surgical fees, for a partially reimbursed insurance—cataract (*See* paragraph 3.3.5, Preoperative evaluation, page 97).

Out-patient surgery must not be confused with ambulatory surgery. Indeed, the latter requires "beds" for its external care (in-patients) according to French social security.

In French eye centers (hospitals, clinics), health insurance manages cataract surgery (hardly ever excluded beyond 60 years old) on the basis of conventional price (140 €), patient having to pay extras for premium IOLs.

Additional cost for premium multifocal IOL is at the expense of the patient by virtue of a "peculiar fee requirement" (Art. L 162-22-6 of the French public health Code "Code de la santé publique").

In the scope of a clear lens extraction, so-called Prelex (*PREsbyopic Lens Exchange*), is a non-refund surgery and at own expense for the patient. He will cost few thousand Euros according to eye centers.

Candidates for Prelex surgery are often:
- at least 60 years old,
- with normal visual acuity corrected under high and low contrast,
- with satisfactory resistance to dazzle, and
- ready to pay extras for a phakolaser technique (LenStar™ for example).

If IOL remains an excellent compensating option for hyperopes, moderate hyperopic presbyopes (less then +2.25 diopters) could be an excellent indication of conductive keratoplasty (CK).

This is one of the methods approved by the FDA in the United States for surgical compensation of hyperopia and presbyopia, but France has not been convinced yet.

Nevertheless, its simplicity and relative safety makes it an interesting approach.

3.3.10 Conductive Keratoplasty (CK) (Fig. 3.20)

The principle of CK is simple: it is a controlled concentrical multilocular application of a thermal probe; the probe's radiofrequency of 350 kHz triggers, as a biochemical reaction, a contraction of corneal collagen, which tends to arch the center of the cornea inducing multifocality.

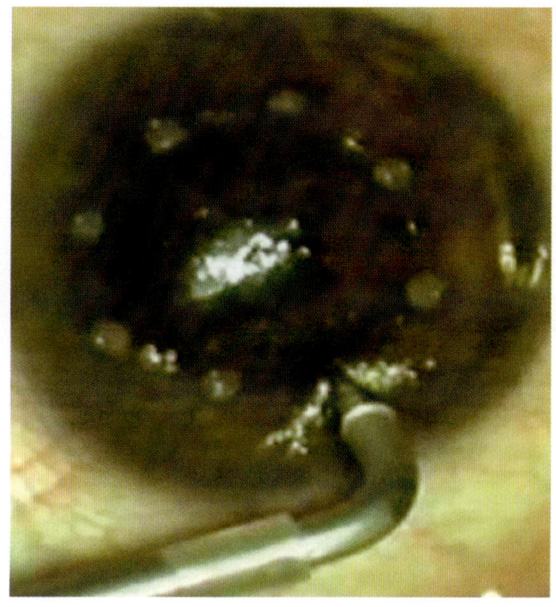

Fig. 3.20 Plotted spots immediately consecutive to CK on a healthy cornea in a presbyopic hyperopia

The shrinkage of the corneal collagen secondary to CK procedure induces a compensation of hyperopia and presbyopia temporarily.

Energetic flow spreads:
- over a thickness of 500 μm from ever epithelialized corneal surface,
- as regularly as possible ("light touch" technique),
- via a probe of 90 μm diameter, and
- with a thermal effect heating the stromal tissues up to 65°C (corneal collagen denaturation and contraction) (Fig. 3.21).

Microscopically speaking, CK process induces the contraction at the level of a stromal cylinder:
- of 100 μm diameter by 500 μm height,
- perpendicular to the surface, and
- that is distributed in a crown shape with paracentral cornea constriction and arching of the corneal apex.

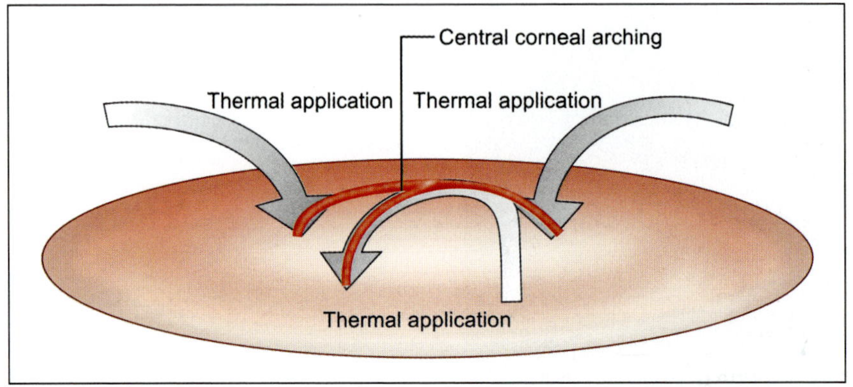

Fig. 3.21 Increasing of the corneal curvatures (bold lines), secondary curvatures coming after the thermal application (gray arrows) in corneal thickness by CK

The process of the surgery presents a favorable learning curve. It is realized under topical anesthesia, after epithelial markings of the spots laid out on the rings. Rings have diameters of 6, 7 and 8 mm, 8 spots per ring.

Nomogram indicates the number of spots to apply, with the probe perpendicular to the corneal surface, disposed without excessive pressure (*light touch*):

- 16 spots for a correction between +1.00 and +1.75,
- 24 spots between +1.75 and +2.25 diopters.

Procedure may induce astigmatism, voluntarily (correcting a pre-existing low astigmatism) or involuntarily (induction of a non-existent astigmatism prior to surgery):

- if epithelial marking is inaccurate (low visibility or ink excess),
- if the application of the spots is irregular (the probe must remain perpendicular to the corneal surface during all the spot application), and
- or if the probe is inserted more than once at the same place.

In our experiment, CK has short-term good results, but later (2 years) regression is observed in most of the operated patients.

Postoperative pain is significant and the patients often need analgesic and anxiolytic drugs, above all in case of bilateral procedure.

After 6 months, 1% of the eyes have lost one distal visual acuity line but most read Jaeger 1. After 12 months, no eye had a loss superior to 2 lines with a visual acuity superior to 20/10 in distant vision, but Jaeger 3 in near vision.

In spite of mitigated results, most of patients (especially hyperopes) claim an improvement of their vision quality in 98% of cases, 84% of whom are satisfied with the intervention and 100% having their distance assessment preserved.

Good candidates for CK correspond to the followings:
- at least 45 years old,
- presbyopia demanding lens or spectacles compensation,
- normal distal visual acuity (sphere inferior to +0.75 diopter in both eyes),
- astigmatism inferior to 0.75 diopter in both eyes without corneal pathology, with normal topography, and
- keratopachymetry superior to 550 μm on the optical zone of 6 mm diameter.

If, CK is reserved for low hyperopia, the intracorneal rings (ICRs) are indicated for young presbyopes presenting low to intermediate myopia reversible monovision.

3.3.11 Intracorneal Rings (ICRs)

Models are INTACS for *INTrACorneal Segments*, KERARING, Keratacx or Ferrara rings (Fig. 3.22).

Broadly speaking, ICRs are the surgical equivalent of the orthokeratological lenses that we have described earlier (*See* paragraph 3.2.4, Orthokeratology, page 92).

The positioning of the ICRs is simple, but the surgical realization may sometimes be a challenge on thin and fragile corneas (Fig. 3.23):
- introduction in the corneal stroma,
- of two polymethylmethacrylate hemi-rings,
- between 300 μm and 450 μm thick,
- with an arch length of 150° (more or less),
- over 80% of the corneal surface, and
- by means of diamond-knife microincision and two femtosecond laser hemidissections (former manual dissection) (Fig. 3.22).

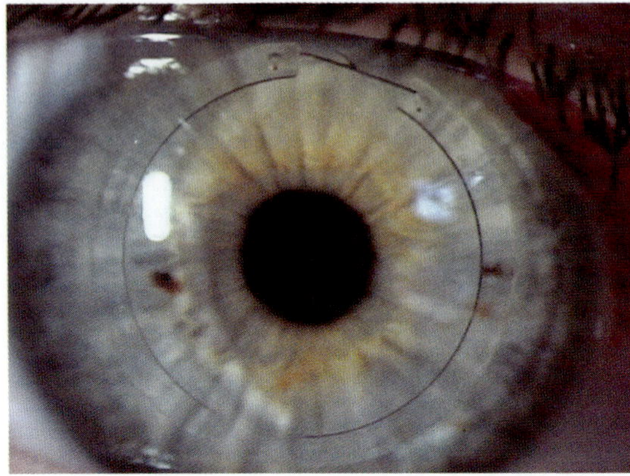

Fig. 3.22 ICRs perfectly centered on the pupil and burried knot in place on the incision (Personal iconography taken from a Rodenstock 5000 slit lamp mounted with a CCD camera)

ICRs implie the central flattening of the cornea and circular bulging corresponding to the rings. This peripheral irregularity induces a multifocal cornea enabling a certain degree of presbyopic correction in myopia.

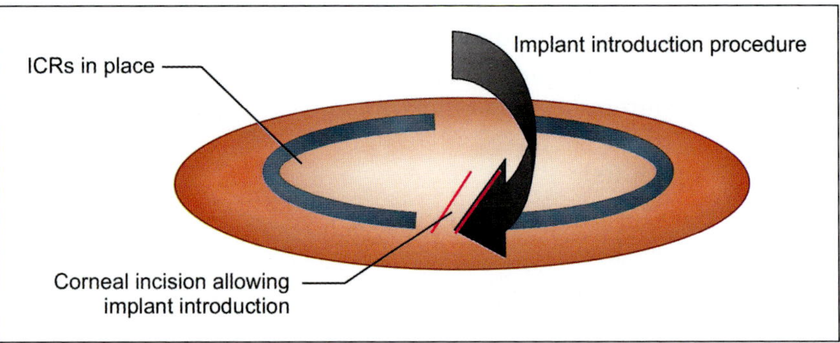

Fig. 3.23 Schematical introduction procedure of two ICRs in the corneal tunnels

Regarding the regularity of the intrastromal cutting as much as the sharpness in the stromal depth, the FS laser allows this technique to find naturally its place in refractive compensations surgical armamentarium.

The presence of both hemi-rings has the role to flatten the central cornea biomechanically, which gradually accentuates, along with corneal wound healing.

To customize the treatment is one of the great advantages this technique offers. The size of the introduced segments modulates the customization, aided with the firm's monogram.

ICRs thus can be replaced to:

- increase myopical correction (in case of lack of optical compensation), or on the contrary, and
- reduce the compensatory effect (with the objective to increase the residual myopia) for facilitating near vision on one eye (*See* paragraph 3.3.2, Monovision, page 95).

ICRs can compensate myopia until about –5.00 diopters, with or without associated astigmatism.

Results are excellent, even though their foreseeable nature is relative and the definitive refractive result evaluated after the sixth postoperative week.

INTACS, Keratacx, KERARINGs are essentially indicated for normal or ectatic corneas (irregular astigmatism). The different shapes and sizes of rings enable to control the antiastigmatogenous effect, with a lesser effect on the residual sphere: as with Ferrara's rings implanted near the center of the cornea.

Contraindications are linked with the existence of a scar or a keratoleptynsis (localized corneal thinning) likely to cause preoperative complications such as perforation:

- of corneal endothelium (in the deepest stromal plane dissections) or,
- of corneal epithelium (in the too superficial corneal dissections).

The long-term tolerance is good, even if a whitish deposit usually surrounds ICRs, without any pejorative meaning appearing, a few months after surgery.

In case of:

- infection of stromal tunnel,
- segment extrusion, or
- excessive deposit.

The simple removal of ICRs permits, most of the time, to come back to the corneal original state. This surgery match with using the other surgical techniques [LASIK (*See* paragraph 3.3.6, Keratosurgecal lasers, page 100), IOLs (*See* paragraph 3.3.9, Lenticular surgeries, page 109)].

3.3.12 Intrastromal Relaxing Femtolaser-mediated Corneal Incisions (IntraCOR) (Fig. 3.24)

As we saw it (*See* paragraph 3.3, page 93), femtosecond laser represents one of the most innovative tools in refractive surgery field.

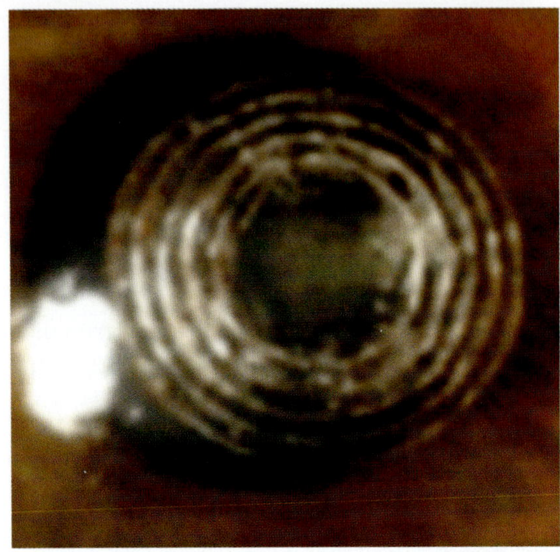

Fig. 3.24 Multiple circumferential intrastromal circles just after intraCOR femtolaser application

IntraCOR is performed on the non-dominant eye to provide a multifocal cornea compensating presbyopia in emmetropia and low hyperopia.

Since the beginning of 2007, Argentinian Antonio RUIZ proposes innovative solution to compensate presbyopia by intracorneal photodisruption with FS laser.

Intrastromal incisions exert relaxing effect.

These incisions are not connected with the corneal anterior and posterior surfaces.

The aim is to create hyper-prolate deformation (*See also* paragraph 2.5.6.5, Corneal asphericity and OA, page 78) of the central cornea without neither making the tissue slimmer nor opening the corneal surface, which is close to conductive keratoplasty (*See* paragraph 3.3.11, Intracorneal rings (ICRs), page 125).

This more minimalist laser approach has been evaluated. It does consist in inducing a certain level of corneal pseudo-accommodation, by creating negative corneal asphericity (*See also* paragraph 2.5.6.1, Aberrometry, page 69) that a myopical minimal shift compensates. It explains the refractive stability in emmetropes (Fig. 3.25).

Thanks to a curvature flattening, laser makes a dozen of concentrical rings in the central 3 to 5 mm.

The procedure takes place on the pupil, lasts less than 30 seconds and short-term results are impressive. The procedure is only perfomed on non-dominant eye.

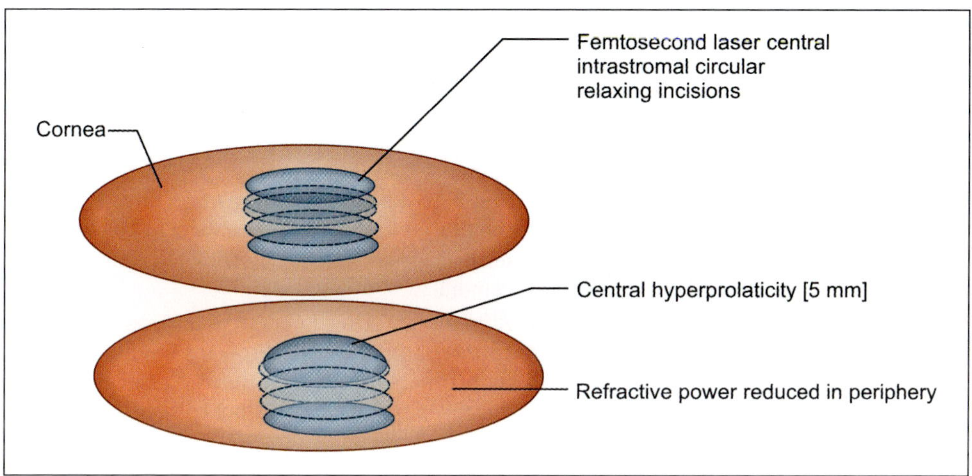

Fig. 3.25 Schematic diagram of intraCOR action process

3.3.13 Radial Keratotomy (RK) (Fig. 3.26)

Let us mention, for the record, a myopic keratosurgery historical technique that the coming of the excimer laser techniques ousted in the 90s: the Radial Keratotomy (RK).

Radial keratotomy is an old technique, but efficient, which consisted in disposing many preperforating radial corneal incisions that:

- we can control according to a nomogram,
- from the limbus towards the center (centripetal) or from the center towards the limbus (centrifugal),
- calibrated deep down,
- carried out with diamond-knife, and
- sparing a central optical zone superior to 3 mm diameter.

This technique was really appreciated for low and moderate myopic optical compensation. In high myopia, there is a risk of exceeded number of radial incisions to excess leading to corneal decompensation (Fig. 3.26).

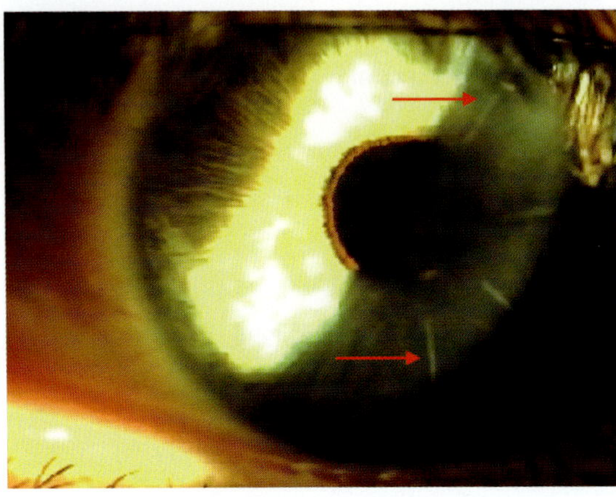

Fig. 3.26 Radial keratotomy (red arrows) as performed in the 80s for low or moderate myopia (Personal iconography taken from a Rodenstock 5000 slit lamp mounted with a CCD camera)

Although effective in correcting myopia, RK has proved the spontaneous evolution toward mild or severe hyperopia with time. Operated patients have been suffering from increased presbyopia without correction.

The relevant setting of the incisions, the control of mini-RK (respecting limbus) or, on the contrary, the sclerolimbal keratotomy (limbus extending into adjacent sclera) did prove themselves. From our own experience, at the age of presbyopia added with the corneal handling of low or moderate myopia, success was measured with:

- distant vision,
- intermediate vision (multifocality between the corneal incisions), and
- near vision (accommodative effect), (*See also* paragraph 4.1, Presbyopia and accommodative relaxation surgeries, page 137).

The clinical evolution in the operated patients has confirmed hyperopic tendency that compromises initial good result. These unsatisfied patients may now consider more stable recent techniques [LASIK (*See* paragraph 3.3.7, PresbyLASIK, page 103), IOLs (*See* paragraph 3.3.9, Lenticular surgeries, page 109)].

Cornea is an outstanding area for presbyopia optical compensation. It has recently benefited from interesting innovations: intracorneal inlays.

3.3.14 Intracorneal Inlays

Inlays are hydrophilic soft contact lenses we place within the central corneal thickness. We put them into a corneal flap perfomed with microkeratome or femtosecond laser (LASIK method, *See* paragraph 3.3.6, Keratosurgical lasers, page 100).

Three types of inlays are now used with optical properties.

1. Refractive effect-zone shape inlay (Flexivue Microlens™):
   - small diameter (3.2 mm),
   - permits to vault the central cornea arch and to correct hyperopias until +5.00 diopters, apparently with less sharpness than LASIK,
   - Hydrophilic acrylic polymer,
   - 1.6 mm diameter central plane perforated disc,
   - annular refractive peripheral zone (addition +0.25 to +3.50 diopters), and
   - specific injector for an optical placement (provided by Presbia corp).

   The implant may benefit later from the clinical developments of anisometropia, likely to generate corneal multifocality (*See* paragraph 3.3.7, PresbyLASIK, page 103).

2. Index refractive effect inlay (Vue+™):
   - slip under a corneal flap, at 30% of corneal thickness,
   - the centrocorneal position triggers central addition.

   Modifying the corneal anterior curvature in the 3 mm zone, this implant may not give all clinical benefits if not exactly centered (transparency due to similar refringence index to cornea n=1.376). We should develop them to multizone, multifocal inlays, to pretend real presbyopic compensation. Inlays profiles:
   - 2 mm diameter,
   - 78% hydrophilic hydrogel, and
   - 30 µm thick in the center, 5 µm thick in the periphery.

3. Stenopeic-effect inlay (Kamra™):
   - allows to increase depth of field,
   - is a 3.8-millimeter diameter ring-shaped small item (8,400 microholes),
   - gets a 1.6-millimeter central circular aperture as stenopeic hole (*See also* paragraph 1.3.2, Miosis, page 13),
   - non-transparent microperforated for micro surgical facility, and
   - 5 µm thick.

The surface of the disk is microperforated to also allow a better tissue biointegration, and the lenticule must be exactly facing the entry pupil, under a LASIK flap. The Acu Target Surgical Unit enhances the proper placement with the 3D eyetracker system.

Consequently, Kamra inlay does not base action principle on either multifocality, or defocusing, but upon increasing the clearness zone on both sides of intermediate vision (field depth) (*See also* paragraph 1.3.2, Miosis, page 13).

Nearly all of the operated presbyopic patients can read with 20/20 in farsightedness and Jaeger 1 in nearsightedness after one year.

Initial corneal edema usually regresses in a few days. However, the major risk is the short-term secondary decentration after implantation.

With large pupils, the patients (95%) often suffer from halos and slightly lower contrast sensitivity.

Epikeratophakia is an historical corneal inlay developed to compensate aphakia or high hyperopia:
- not synthetic natural cornea from a postmortem donor,
- its shape is modified to obtain meniscus lens with adequate power to correct hyperopia, and
- implanted under corneal flap.

This is the oldest refractive surgery we have known, which the Colombian surgeon J Barraquer initiated. He is the father of lamellar refractive surgery.

We can imagine that the historical keratophakic intracorneal lens might be updated for emmetropic presbyopes or hyperopes.

The present simplicity of the corneal flap realization with whether FS laser or microkeratome, the insertion of a hydrogel or plastic lenticule, under the flap is an attractive method.

We call corneal lenticule a synthetic lamella that is:
- transparent and biocompatible,
- likely to play a refractive effect, and
- in the stromal lamellae of the cornea.

Thanks to their efficiency, corneal lenticules might then compete with IOLs (*See* paragraph 3.3.9, Lenticular surgeries, page 109), CK (*See* paragraph 3.3.10, Conductive keratoplasty (CK), page 122), or intra-COR (*See* paragraph 3.3.12, Intrastromal relaxing femto-mediated corneal incisions (IntraCOR), page 127).

Laser refractive keratosurgery is optimized for myopic subjects because it consists of tissular substraction surgery, which is more difficult to realize for hyperopes: the technique demands to remove twice the amount of corneal tissue per diopter compared to myopic patients (Figs 3.29A and B).

Some reckon that corneal ablation is so important compared with its mixed result (increasing the spherical aberration), that hyperopic excimer laser ablative surgery is rather an absurdity to them.

With intracorneal inlay technique, the setting of the lenticule in the stromal interface changes corneal curvature, without either thinning it up, or taking any corneal tissue out.

Reversibility is total since surgeon only has to lift the flap again **(Figs 3.27 and 3.28)**, take the lenticule out of the interface and put the corneal flap back in place. We cannot conceive this reversibility with LASIK techniques (*See* paragraph 3.3.7, PresbyLASIK, page 103).

The advantage to use these lenticules in presbyopes is reversibility at slit lamp during consultation (according to certain american authors), which is not the case for accommodative IOLs, for instance.

Slit lamp is the basic biomicroscope of all ophthalmological consultation. All intervention with slit lamp exempts us from having recourse to surgical requirements under the operating theater microscope.

Another advantage of corneal lenticules on IOLs is the possibility to exactly position the implant, which is not possible with IOLs going inside the capsular bag.

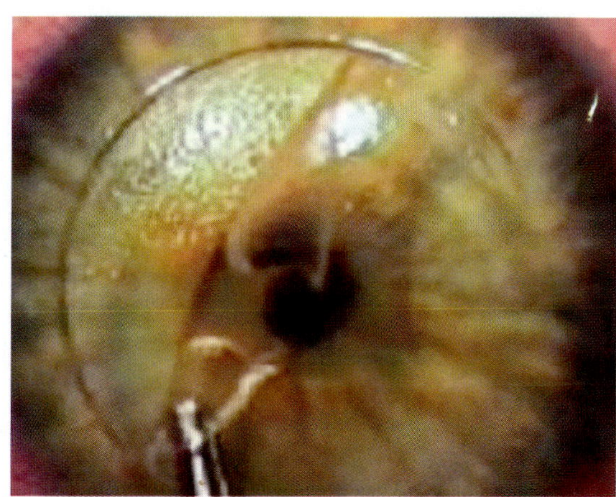

Fig. 3.27 Corneal flap reclined with the forceps after femtolaser application prior to keratorefractive procedure

LASIK flap may be performed with the microkeratome (blade) or laser (light). In the stromal bed under the flap an inlay may be implanted with refractive property.

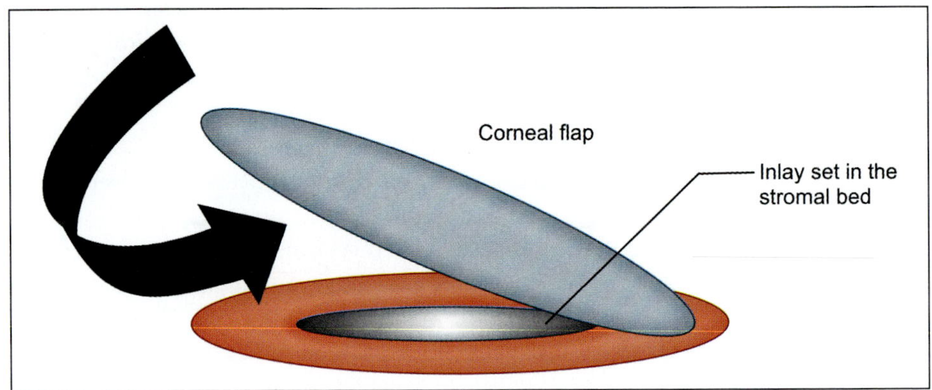

Fig. 3.28 Corneal inlay surgical principle (intrastromal lenticule)

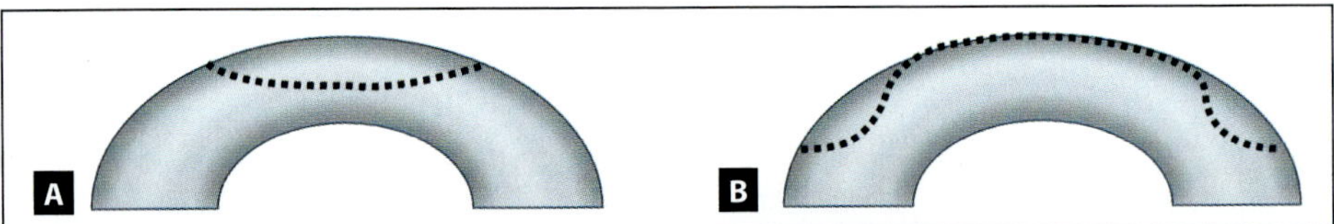

Figs 3.29A and B Refractive keratosurgery profiles of excimer laser photoablation for myopia (A) and hyperopia (B)

Along with the usual insertion procedure to put these intracorneal lenticulas under a LASIK flap, some authors propose to insert the lenticule in an intrastromal pocket (RELEX procedure):

- thanks to a pair of stromal tunnels,
- at a depth of 200 μm each,
- with width of 2.5 millimeter (to let the lenticule go in its 5-millimeter-transversal diameter).

Intrastromal pocket, cut with FS laser presents following advantages:

- no need to use microkeratome,
- avoids cutting complications (free flap, microribs, epithelial invagination (Fig. 3.30), interstitial diffuse lamellar keratitis), and
- prevents any lenticule secondary dislocation.

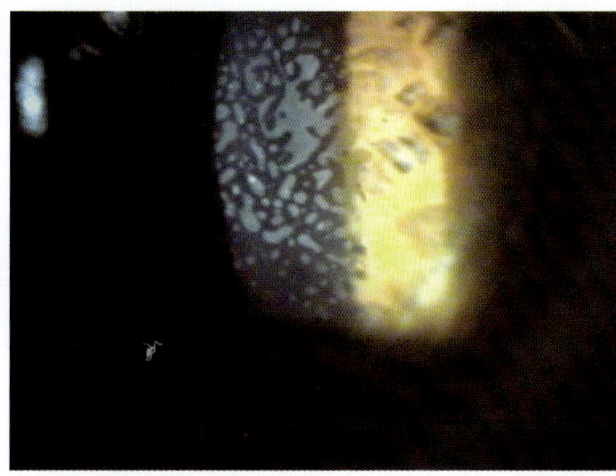

Fig. 3.30 Area of epithelial invagination under a LASIK flap (Personal iconography taken from a Rodenstock 5000 slit lamp mounted with a CCD camera)

Epithelial invagination is the spontaneous migration of epithelium to fill the blind space left between stroma and flap. This disorder must be wiped away if corneal melting appears inducing astigmatism and irregularity of the corneal surface.

A lenticule injector, especially developed to that end, enables to position it within intrastromal pocket (*See* above, page 131).

Indicated for presbyopic hyperopes between +1.00 and +6.00 diopters:

- 6-months checking shows a 5/10 distal visual acuity that is not corrected in most of patients,
- manifest refraction spherical equivalent average is –0.31 diopter,
- refractive unpredictability is inferior to 0.5 diopter in 60% of the patients and inferior to 1 diopter in 90%,
- none of the patients lose more than two lines with this technique.

Brand new intracorneal inlay techniques shows its perfect reversibility and easy implementation.

Still, we need to stand back for a while. On the one hand, we have to judge lenticule biomaterial and long-term perfect tolerance, on the other hand, to check on the long-term preservation of the corneal clearness, in the intrastromal implant vicinity (like deposits with intracorneal rings) (*See* paragraph 3.3.11, Intracorneal rings (ICRs), page 125).

Hence, all these surgical techniques to compensate presbyopia do not restore accommodation.

Furthermore, there are various propositions of scleral techniques in order to restore accommodation.

We will then see if the actual knowledge of accommodation, and the presbyopic residual function, allow us to hope for a true crystalline lens or pseudo-crystalline lens accommodative restoration.

CHAPTER 4

Presbyopia and Accommodative Restoration

While previously studying Helmholtz' classical theory (*See also* paragraph 1.5.1, History, page 28), we have learnt that the zonular laxity induced by the ciliary muscle, generates:

- crystalline lens anterior capsule vaulting and
- increase in refractive power during accommodation.

More recently, Schachar suggested, on the contrary, that the contraction of the ciliary muscle would lead to its expansion outwards, tensing the equatorial radial zonular fibers with concomitant relaxation of the anterior and posterior fibers during accommodation (*See also* paragraph 1.5.2, Experimental modelization, page 30).

Consequently, there would be:

- tension of the anterior crystalloid and,
- arching of the anterior central surface of the crystalline lens (at the expense of a peripheral flattening), responsible for refractive power rise.

Many studies, in particular Adrian Glasser's team, have not validated this new theory (*See also* paragraph 1.5.3, Clinical approach, page 32).

Nonetheless, due to the crystalline lens growth with aging, the distance between crystalline lens equator and ciliary muscle loses 10 μm each year. We have then identified this as one of the probable factors of presbyopia evolution. At the moment, it serves as a foundation for relaxation or supraciliary scleral expansion additive methods (Fig. 4.1).

Relaxation techniques make a passive scleral expansion possible, under intraocular pressure such as:

- anterior ciliary sclerotomy (ACS) (*See* paragraph 4.1.1, Blade anterior ciliary sclerotomy (ACS), page 138) and

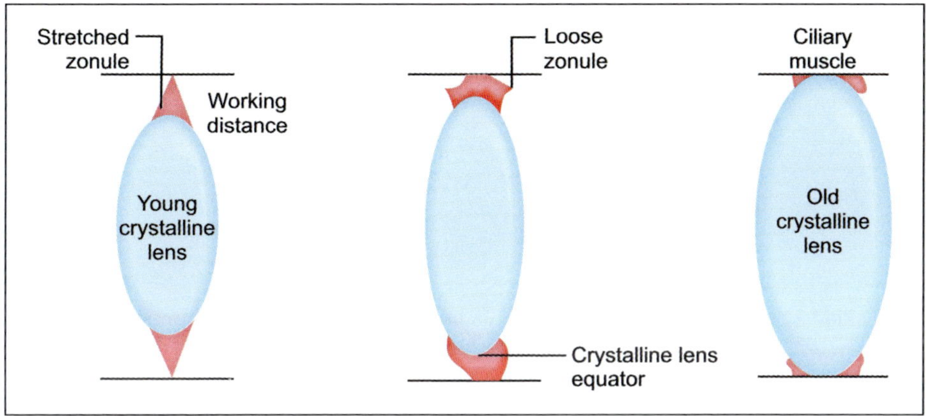

Fig. 4.1 Schematical representation of effects due to crystalline lens growth on zonule fibers in presbyopic evolution according to Schachar's theory

- associated techniques (*See* paragraph 4.1.2, ACS implant, page 139 and paragraph 4.1.3, ACS laser, page 140).

Additive techniques permit an active scleral expansion (potentializing the pressure expansive effect):
- by external ways, using,
    - scleral expansion bands (SEB) (*See* paragraph 4.2.1, Scleral Expansion Bands (SEBs), page 142) or,
    - supraciliary segments or,
- ab interno such the ciliary-zonular tension ring implantation (*See* paragraph 4.4.5, Patented invention of CZTR, page 179).

    We may associate relaxation scleral technique with additive scleral one to increase efficiency with time. Let us develop these different techniques in details.

4.1 PRESBYOPIA AND ACCOMMODATIVE RELAXATION SURGERIES (FIG. 4.2)

Initially, Thornton (*See* Fig. 4.29) found out limbal incisions were connected with accommodation. Indeed, back in the RK days (*See also* paragraph 3.3.13, Radial keratotomy (RK), page 129), he noticed that the

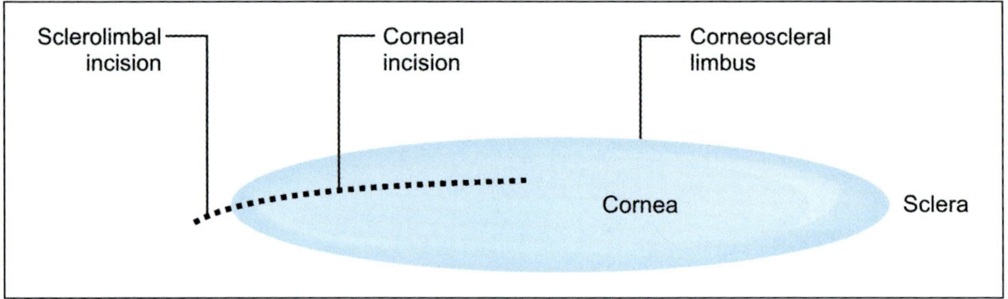

Fig. 4.2 Diagram of a corneoscleral RK likely to play a part in accommodation by inducing a scleral expansion (superior oblique view)

realization of centripetal or centrifugal incisions, widely encroaching on the limbus and adjacent sclera, contributed to a preserved accommodation in operated myopes.

He deducted that, on top of corneal topographical modification linked with the RK, the extended incisions beyond the sclerocorneal limbus could influence accommodation.

4.1.1 Blade Anterior Ciliary Sclerotomy (ACS) (Fig. 4.3)

Hypothetically, sclerotomies regularly distributed before the anterior part of the ciliary body namely, anterior ciliary sclerotomy (ACS), had the tendency to exert a relaxing effect on the adjacent sclera, appearing as scleral vaulting. The ultrabiomicroscopical observation of the incised sclera confirmed this hypothesis.

From 1990, Thornton (*See* Fig. 4.29) published his first favorable clinical results about the accommodative plane, immediately gaining from 1 to 2.50 diopters.

So as to increase its efficiency, Thornton proposed to double the sclerotomies in each quadrant, at a calibrated depth of 600 µm and to realize it with a diamond-knife.

Data in the scientific literature about ACS confirmed my personal experience:
* depends on the subjects and varies from 1 to 2.50 diopters,
* immediate (from the day after operation), but unfortunately,

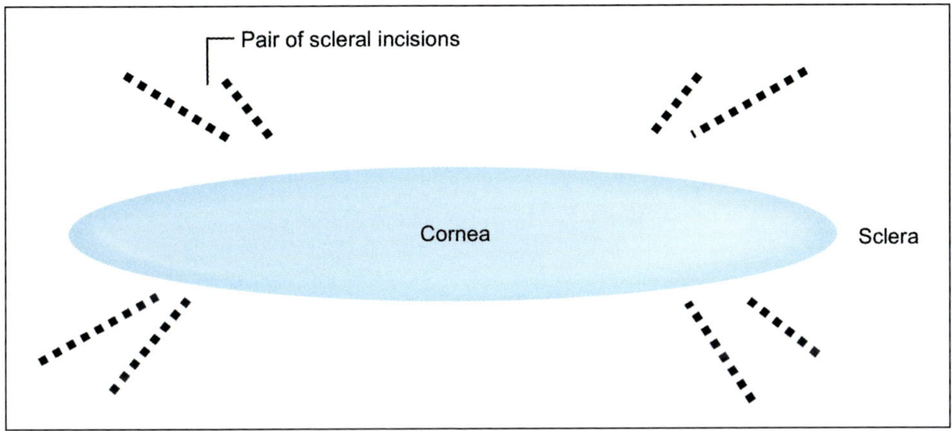

Fig. 4.3 Schematical representation of four pairs of ACS on a superior oblique view

- of short duration (between 2 and 4 months, in my series), after what all the subjects totally lose the accommodative gain in less than one year.

Immediate side effects are connected with the incision depth and length, causing spontaneously resolutive subconjunctival hemorrhages.

Side effects and complications are transitory hyphema, not to say expulsive choroidal hemorrhage with or without choroid hernia.

4.1.2 ACS Implant

To delay the ACS accommodative effects, in 1998, Fukasaku (*See* Fig. 4.29) proposed to realize:
- four pairs of retrolimbal radial incisions,
- 95% deep in the scleral thickness determined with UBM (*See* paragraph 4.2.2, Accommodative IOLs, page 146),
- with suture of a silicone implant to keep the incision open, the implant being supposed to control scleral wound healing, hence stabilizing accommodative result.

The accommodative gain is around an average of 1.9 diopter, with stable results for 6 months.

Unfortunately, the absence of ulterior data, let us believe the silicone implants are unable to control the intrascleral wound healing that comes with the extrusion of the material and long-term accommodative inefficiency.

Wrongfully thinking silicone-made implants could contribute to a premature healing of anterior ciliary sclera, in 2002, Jory proposed the implantation of a titanium device in the scleral incisions, with no more success.

4.1.3 ACS Laser

Other authors, like Lin, reversely thought that the nature of the scleral incision itself could compromise the postoperative wound healing and the regressive results in terms of accommodative gain. In 1998, he thus presented a scleral incision technique (Fig. 4.4):

- without using the diamond-knife but,
- with a YAG Erbium laser,
    - 3 µm long wave (limitation of thermal effect),
    - delivering spots of 400 µm through an optical fiber and a contact cone,
    - according to a surgical procedure called *laser assisted presbyopia reversal* (LAPR).

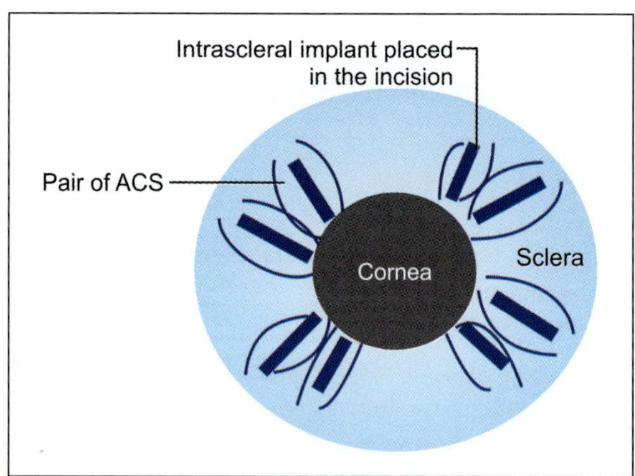

Fig. 4.4 Scheme of eight sclerotomies implants placed in the gaping incisions (front view)

However, the photoablative principle of the lasers developed for scleral (wavelength of 3000 nm) or corneal surgery (wavelength 1093 nm) remains unchanged, these lasers tackle collagens of very different nature.

During surgical process, a pair of radial incisions is realized:
- of 4.5 mm length,
- separated by a 2.5 mm space,
- 80% deep of the sclera,
- 0.5 mm at the posterior part of the limbus,
- in each quadrant.

An international study on LAPR gave immediate favorable results:
- with very fast visual rehabilitation (1 hour),
- with no complications, and
- still satisfactory after 6 months with 93% of patients reading Jaeger 2 and 100% having accommodation superior to 1 diopter (between 1.00 and 3.25 diopters, 2.4 diopters as an average).

The final result of LAPR is an increase in scleral circumferential diameter of about 10 mm (Fig. 4.5).

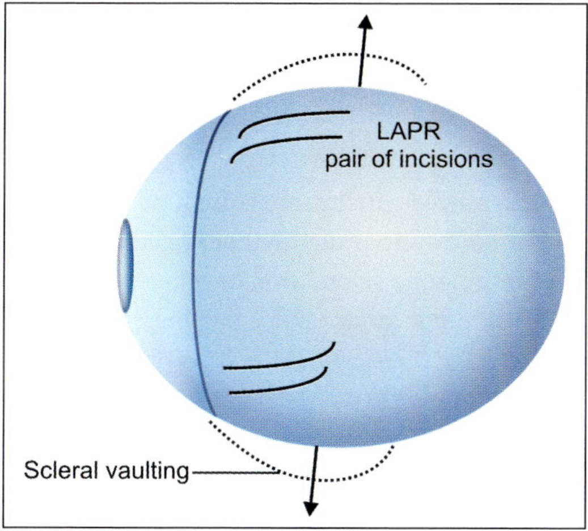

Fig. 4.5 Increase in circumferential diameter by scleral vaulting under LAPR relaxing incisions (lateral view of the eyeball)

The cooperation of the patients who have been operated on this technique was of paramount importance and required regular reading training every hour.

Results after 24 months were excellent since:
- all the patients seemed able to read Jaeger 1,
- most of the patients have seen their farsightedness slightly improved, whereas
- intermediate vision was still excellent.

A synthetical collagen matrix:
- would allow a scleral protection for the comfort and that,
- would prevent wound healing (tissue recolonization) and the regression of the refractive effect,
- is under development.

4.2 PRESBYOPIA AND IMPLANT ACCOMMODATIVE SURGERIES

4.2.1 Scleral Expansion Bands (SEBs) (Fig. 4.6)

PMMA bands:
- can be set in,
- at the four cardinal points,
- within a scleral tunnel, realized at the two-third of the ciliary scleral thickness.

Polymethylmethacrylate (PMMA) is a polymerized substance, hard and transparent, with biocompatibility on ocular tissues, which have been proved for many decades.

Their length, their width and the design of SEB have evolved over three generations upto now.

SEBs are to increase the distance between ciliary body and equator (circumlenticular space), working distance (*See* Fig. 4.1 and paragraph 1.5.1, History, page 28) by enlarging the scleral ring itself.

Suggested action lies in stretching sclera (lifting effect), by vaulting anterior ciliary muscle, in order to restore the zonule tension while preserving reversibility.

The term "lifting" indeed conveys the notion of stretching applied on the sclera under the effect of a SEB implantation that a scleral vaulting, visible on the implantation sites, represents (Fig. 4.7).

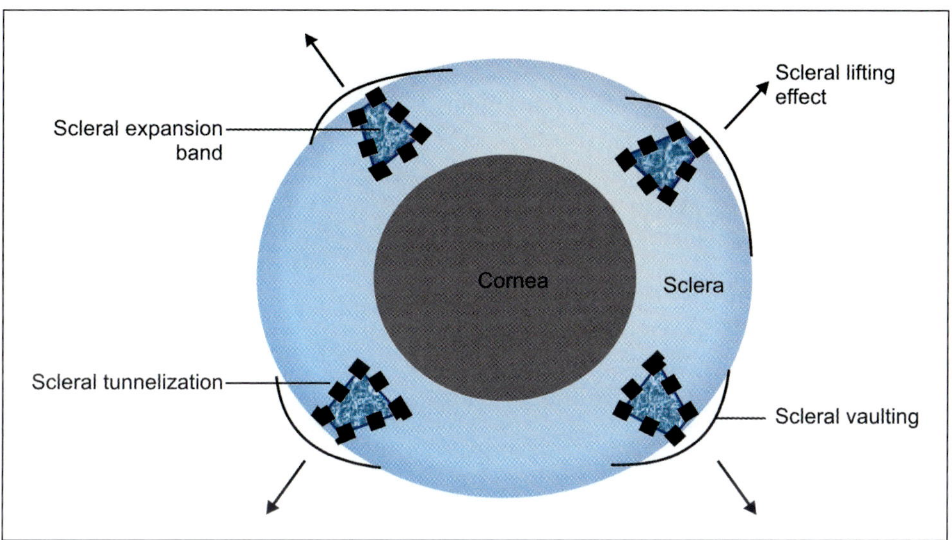

Fig. 4.6 Four SEBs set in scleral tunnels and responsible for scleral lifting and vaulting effects (schematical front view)

American studies have revived the interest in SEBs, their immediate results to correct presbyopia being excellent.

People who received these implants could gain until 7 lines in near visual acuity, with an average of around 3 lines.

Certain results went beyond our expectations, which is rather disturbing.

Scleral PMMA inserts are based upon a refocusing approach, according to which presbyopia, for it is of ectodermal ontological nature, is a product of crystalline lens continuous growth. Besides, these inserts are made to enable presbyopic eyes to focus in near vision, by simply increasing the working distance within circumlenticular space (*See* Fig. 4.1).

When crystalline lens equator grows towards ciliary muscle, equatorial zonule exerts less tension on the muscle (*See* Fig. 4.1).

The decrease in ciliary muscle tension is due to aging and reduces as much the stretching action as its contraction efficiency.

Scleral implanted patients between 50 and 60 years old:
- got all a near visual acuity of Jaeger 3 (J3) and
- demanded a minimal addition of 1.25 diopter for 20/16 near reading equivalent.

Scleral implants (Fig. 4.7):
- rectangular-shaped ones,
- placed through sclera,
- in four anatomical quadrants,
- to expand sclera around the implant.

SEBs tends to increase the expansion with:
- its deformation mechanical effect, and
- the hydraulic effect of pressure on the sclera (towards the inside of the eye).

After 6 months:
- 84% of the implanted patients still read the equivalent of 20/10 Jaeger 4 (J4) and even better on the MNRead card,
- 70% see 20/16 or even better on the Sloan card, and
- 42% preserving a distal angular acuity of at least 20/10 on Landolt C scale.

As for quality, these results got close to:
- multifocal IOLs, or even accommodative ones, and
- the excimer laser corneal techniques.

As opposed to scleral techniques that remains reversible and does not alter distant vision.

Improvement in near vision by this technique is:
- only partial,
- not reproducible, and
- not ever lasting.

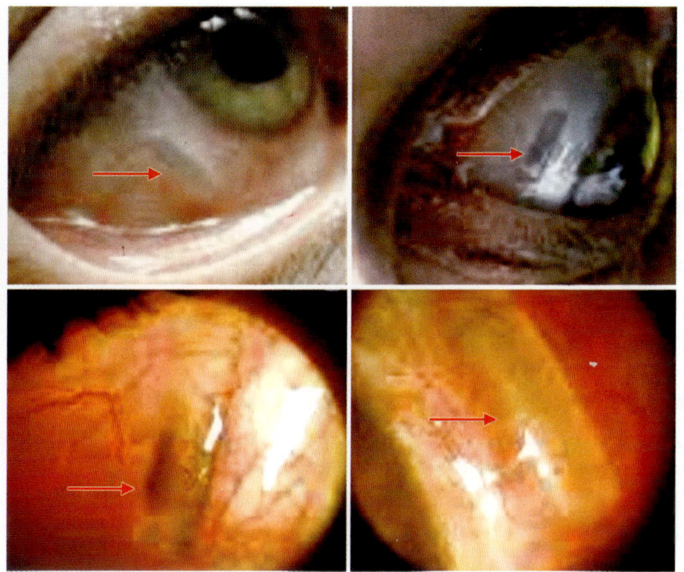

Fig. 4.7 SEBs in place in each quadrant (red arrows) of the eye operated for accommodative restoration in case of presbyopic emmetropia

Rigid PMMA SEBs exerts, when implanted, a lifting effect on scleral surface involving the vaulting of anterior ciliary muscle, therefore an increasing of the internal zonule tension, hence, a restoration of the working distance to improve accommodation.

Moreover, the obtained partial benefit may only be based on a pseudo-accommodation phenomenon (*See also* paragraph 1.5.5, Pseudo-accommodation, page 37) and visual training, particularly explaining that cases of nearsightedness improvement was concerning the non-operated controlateral eye!

Nevertheless, we could observe some complications such as:

- migration,
- extrusion, and even
- scleral necrosis.

In these conditions, despite the efforts that the defensors make to standardize, simplify and secure the SEB surgery by automatizing gesture and adjusting nomogram, it has not broken through.

Along with these scleral techniques, so-called "accommodative" IOLs have developed, too. They are called accommodative since their artificial crystalline lens would be supposed to restore accommodation.

4.2.2 Accommodative IOLs (Figs 4.8A and B)

Together with different systems of IOLs established to restore accommodation, soft connection between haptics and optic allows optic to move anteriorly, during ciliary muscle accommodative contraction and posterior vitreous dynamics (Fig. 4.9).

Clinical results of these IOLs have been a controversial topic. Numerous studies have found out a low transitory and accommodative gain (less than 1 diopter). Others, like us, have found no effect at all upon accommodation.

Theoretical accommodative effect is about 1 diopter per 730 μm anterior moving, meaning that we ought to need a 2.2-millimeter moving to obtain an additive effect of 3 diopters (!).

Capsular bag fibrosis makes such a movement unsure, since it limits the optic moving possibility.

Capsular fibrosis is a wound healing process that naturally settles within the operated capsular bag.
This phenomenon is inescapable, irreversible and source of retraction, rigidifying tissue and leading to opacity (posterior capsular opacification), (*See also* paragraph 3.3.9, Lenticular surgeries, page 109).

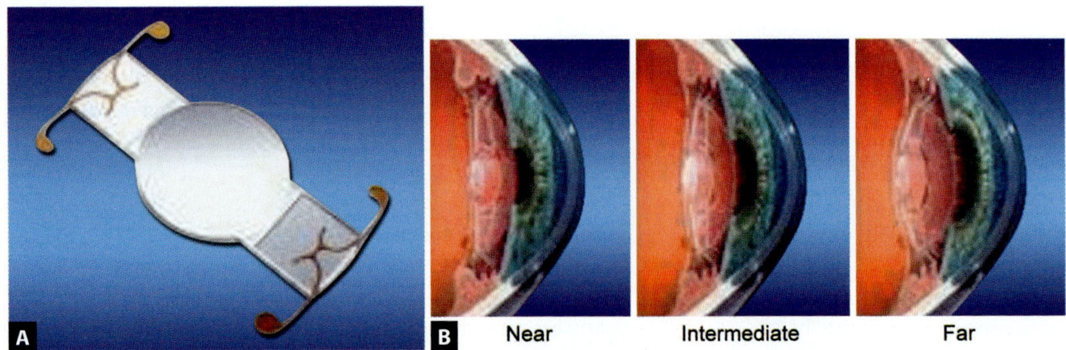

Figs 4.8A and B Accommodative IOL (A) and its mechanism of action (B)

Accommodative IOLs must be implanted with perfect surgery to be sure to get the best results on presbyopia. Patients recently operated need to be dilated in order to have the implant in good position for further dynamic process.

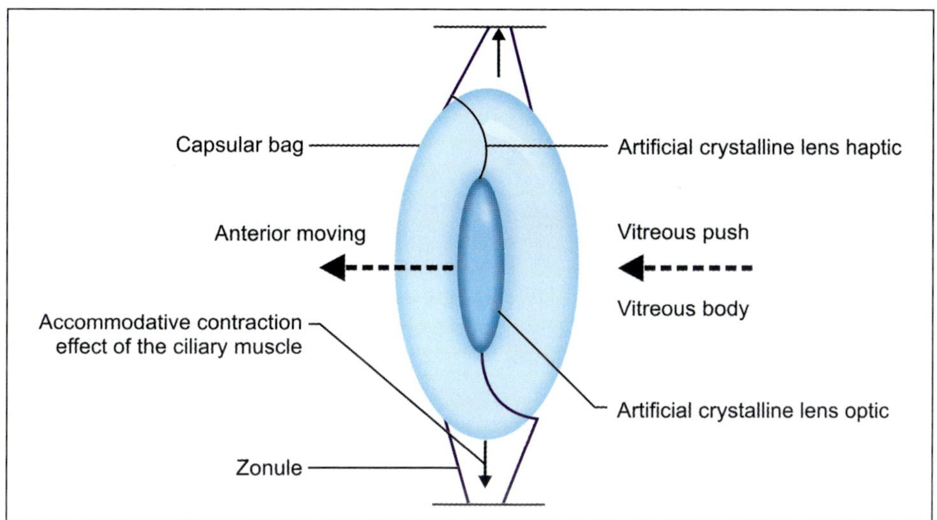

Fig. 4.9 Schematical dynamics of the accommodative IOL in place in the capsular bag (lateral view)

As a matter of fact, a study in ultrabiomicroscopy after pilocarpine instilling has shown:

- an average anterior moving of only 314 µm (that is 0.5 diopter) for some IOLs and
- a slight average backward movement of 50 µm for other implants (!).

Ultrabiomicroscopy (UBM), a bidimensional scanner using ultrasound as a means of immersion and rectilinear scanning, provides us with qualitative and quantitative information on anterior segment structures (*See also* paragraph 1.5.3, Clinical approach, page 32).

The main advantage of UBM exploratory technique is the high axial resolution, although the low penetration in the tissues (Fig. 4.10).

In the scope of accommodative IOLs study, we could obtain with this examination technique a lot of information about relationships between:

- ciliary processes,
- zonule, and
- capsular bag (*See* Fig. 4.25).

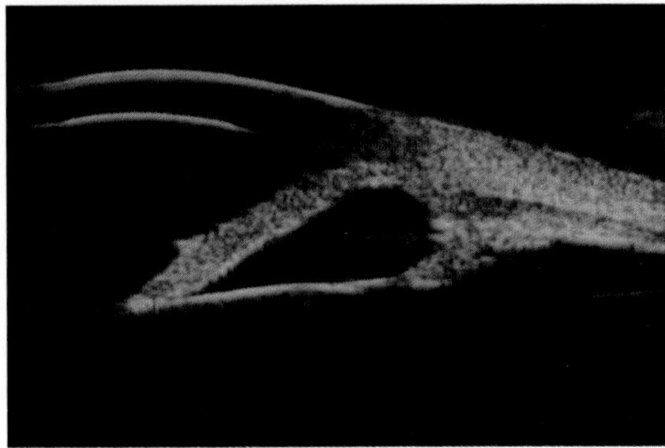

Fig. 4.10 UBM image of the ciliary sulcus (red arrow) between iris root and ciliary body (Personal iconography taken from a UBM probe mounted on a UD6000 Tomey Echograph)

UBM uses ultrasounds (US) for exploring of the soft tissues of the eye. US wave reflects on the liquids of the body but is interrupted in the air.

One of the highest difficulties with this imaging system is to obtain objectively reproducible and reliable measures: when the same observer analyzes and measures with UBM, reliability is excellent.

As a consequence of the subjective nature of the position markers, different observers have less reliability to obtain reliable measures.

As a result, if we measure different images with different operators, the reliability is unacceptable.

Though UBM has accurate biometrical functions, this is not a technique, which can be used for:

- angle-to-angle, or sulcus-to-sulcus measurements,
- visualization of crystalline lens nuclear and posterior portion,
- providing a topographical or pachymetrical map.

With of 50 MHz or 35 MHz probes, we find statistically significant differences before and after accommodative stimuli in measures of:

- camerular angle,
- angle between ciliary processes and sclera, and
- angle between ciliary processes and iris.

In implanted eyes with standard monofocal IOL, UBM analysis demonstrates an accommodative movement of the anterior segment structures.

Crystalline lens surgery induces a rise in anterior chamber depth (around 40 µm).

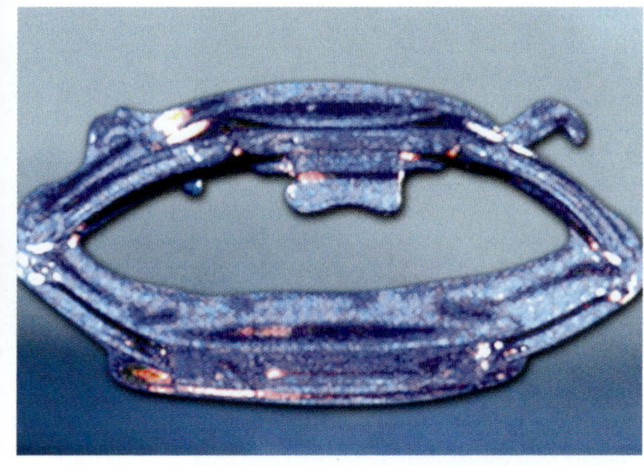

Fig. 4.11 Example of a double-optics IOL for restoring accommodation in presbyopia

Accommodative IOLs use the residual flexibility of the capsular bag to allow changing shape during accommodation, hence changing IOL power for far, near and intermediate vision.

Accommodation stimulus in posterior chamber pseudophake implies:

- sulcus-to-sulcus distance and ciliary ring diameter reduction,
- iris-ciliary processes distance reduction, and
- ciliary processes-iris angle reduction.

Some models of accommodative IOLs are 5° angle closed-loop monoblocks, others have two silicone optics (the anterior optic of 32 diopters is mechanically coupled with the posterior optic of negative power, varying according to the biometry) (Fig. 4.11).

Monoblock IOL is defined as an implant synthetized in one step, using the same material, whether at the level of haptics or optic.

On the contrary, we qualify an implant as two-piece IOL when haptics are secondarily made connected to the optic of often different material (Fig. 4.12).

When ciliary body is at rest, accommodative IOL is focused on distant vision:

- stretched zonule (according to Helmoltz), (*See also* paragraph 1.5.1, History, page 28),
- axial shortening of capsular bag,
- convergence of the two optics, and
- stretching of the spring (Fig. 4.11).

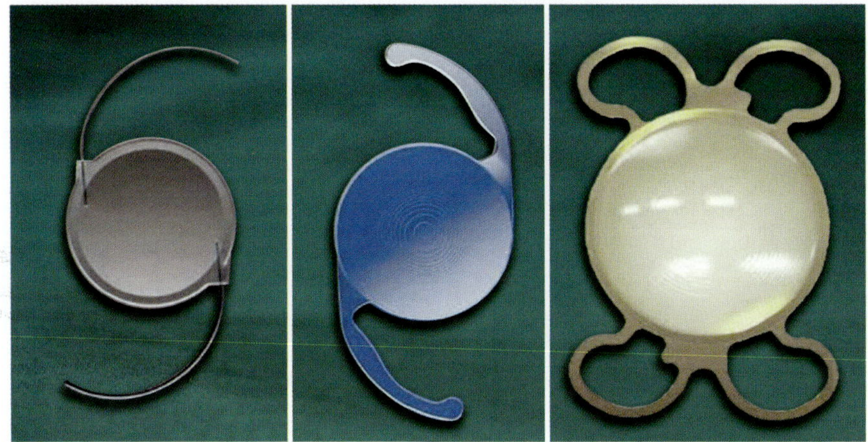

Fig. 4.12 Examples of different designs in IOLs: two-piece (left),
one-piece (monoblock) bipodal (center), monoblock quadripodal (right)

The designs of IOLs are not only important for stability in the eye, but also relevant with an accurate presbyopic surgery, and optimal optical function.

Optic dual lens is made to be inserted into the eye by a 3.6- to 3.8-mm incision in clear cornea.

This soft implant unfolds in the eye and reveals the presence of two optics linked by a spring system.

The 5.5-millimeter diameter anterior optic presents a strong optical power and the 6-mm diameter posterior optic, a lesser one.

The spring activates the anterior optic and modifies near vision focusing to distant vision.

When ciliary muscle is contracted (Fig. 4.13), IOL focuses for the nearsightedness (Schachar's theory):

- relaxed zonule,
- capsular relaxation,
- spring freeing and divergence between the two optics, and
- anterior movement of the anterior optic.

Recent evaluations showed the IOLs still worked correctly a year after implantation.

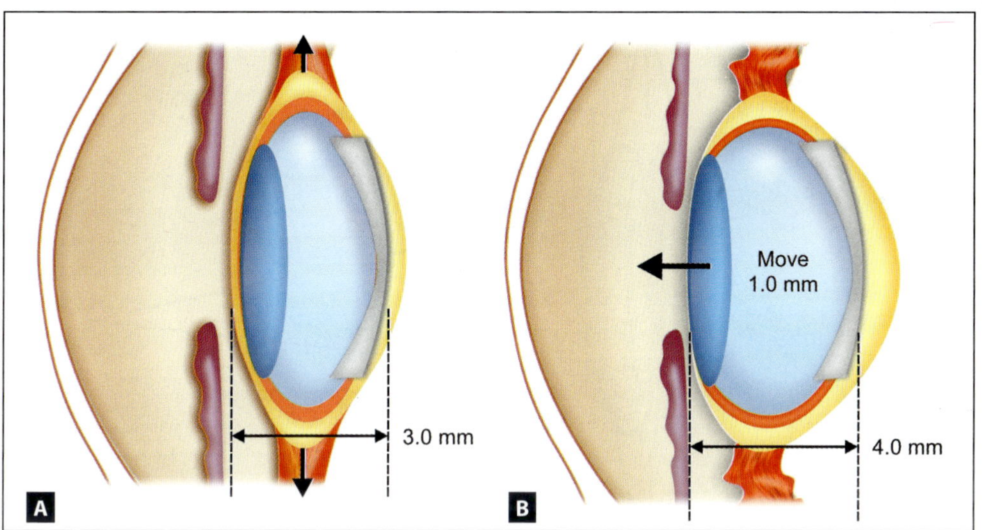

Figs 4.13A and B Schematical dynamics with a two-parts accommodative IOL:
near vision in accommodate state (A), far vision at rest (B)

The special design of this accommodative IOL is based on the accommodative process according to Schachar's theory (opposite to Helmholtz' theory) *(See also* paragraph 1.5, Accommodative etiopathogenesis, page 28).

Accommodative results are satisfactory:
- distant vision superior to 20/10 in 91% of the cases,
- intermediate vision superior to 97%, and
- near vision without additional correction in 84%.
  Reading speed is better compared to a standard implant (160 words/mn versus 23 words/mn).
  Contrasts sensitivity is excellent and there is no perception of any halos.

The very innovative concept of dual optic deserves peculiar attention.

This silicone IOL, made up of two optics (anterior and posterior), is also made interdependent by a spring system. Consequently, the posterior optic remains fixed, applied against the posterior capsule.

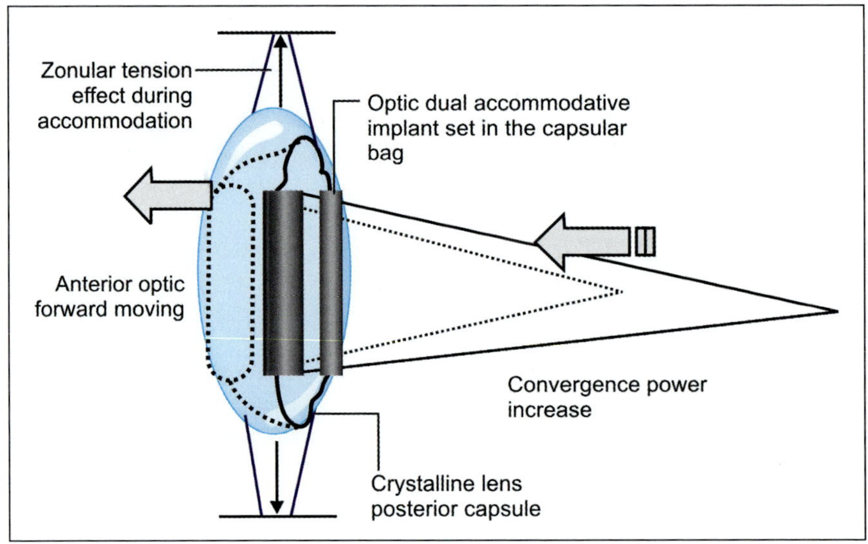

Fig. 4.14 Schematical representation on a side view of the optic dual in capsular bag and during accommodation

The anterior optic, being extremely convergent (32 diopters), can move forward during ciliary muscle contraction.

Accommodative effort goes together with:
- capsular bag contraction,
- anterior vitreous thrust, and
- haptic flexibility.

Even though moving is short, accommodative effect is maximized by the high converging power of the anterior optic.

The posterior optic, the power of which is negative and variable, stays against the posterior capsule during accommodative process (Fig. 4.14).

4.3 OTHER SURGERIES OF ACCOMMODATION

4.3.1 Phakomodulation

To use residual accommodation (*See also* paragraph 1.2.3, Accommodative involution, page 9), other authors, waiting for phako-Ersatz, propose a natural crystalline lens remodeling by phakomodulation.

What we call Ersatz, according to Germanic terminology, is an element replacing some defective or missing item, without being a true and exact copy of the original element.

A phako-Ersatz is thus a substitutive crystalline lens having the same properties as the natural one (*See* Fig. 4.19).

This approach is a matter of modifying the crystalline lens mechanical characteristics. It aims at finding the compliance that an efficient accommodative answer requires, while ciliary muscle contracts or when zonule relaxes.

4.3.1.1 Femtosecond (FS) Laser Lentotomy (Fig. 4.15)

At the moment, we have admitted that the ciliary body keeps contracting at the age of presbyopia and that the capsule remains elastical.

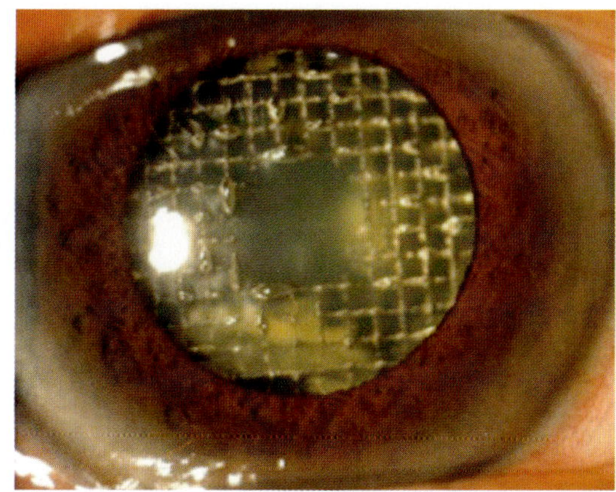

Fig. 4.15 Femtosecond laser lentotomy
Ultraspeed laser is used on crystalline lens to perform accurate microincisions for remodeling or extracting as shown on figure.

Only the crystalline lens becomes denser and harder with aging, so much that the present forces are not powerful enough to deform the crystalline lens.

A German team proposed accommodative restoration by increasing lenticular flexibility. They would proceed by means of laser impulsions handled inside the crystalline lens in order to change its elasticity and its deformability.

FS laser allows to produce intralenticular incisions with great sharpness and without collateral damage thanks to ultrashort laser pulses: lentotomy.

Lentotomy bases its principle on the fact that, if we use laser wavelength close to infrared, both cornea and crystalline lens remain transparent for this radiation.

As a result, we can focus a FS laser:

- inside crystalline lens,
- without open-sky surgery of eyeball, and
- the laser inducing an optical cavitation (*See also* paragraph 3.3.6, Keratosurgerical lasers, page 100).

Moving laser spot inside crystalline lens structure, we may realize a tissue disruption in three dimensions, and thus create a cut-plane.

Animal experiments have confirmed that the application of small laser cuts inside the crystalline lens do not induce short and medium term (3 months) cataract.

So as to give certain elasticity back to crystalline lens, ilaser has been only performed on crystalline lens nucleus by making some gliding planes.

The focal moving of the FS laser impacts entails these planes according to predefined geometric shapes (Fig. 4.16).

Three basic geometric shapes have been tested to create gliding planes.

With the combination of these three shapes the greatest deformability is observed in the crystalline lens, making sure the central area is respected: two arms-of-a-wheel connected by radial, cylindrical corresponding cuts (both cylinders being linked by annular cuts at their anterior and posterior ends) (Fig. 4.16).

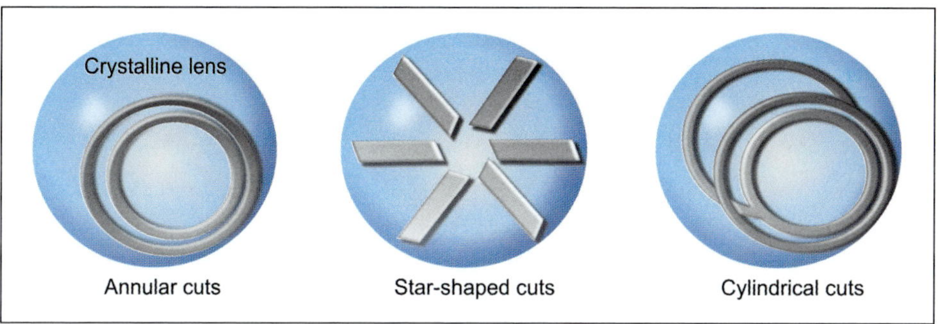

Fig. 4.16 From a side view, schematical examples of FS laser cuts in crystalline lens nucleus, geometrically shaped and likely to restore lenticular accommodation

To test these lentotomized crystalline lenses, they were put at the center of a rotating platform with centrifugal strength proportional to the rotation speed (Fig. 4.17):

- at rest (0 RPM=round per minute),
- 1035 RPM, and
- 1850 RPM.

Centrifugal strength was to simulate the tension exerted by the ciliary muscle in vivo during accommodation (*See* paragraph 4.4.6, Feasibility study, page 186).

High resolution cameras were used to take instantaneous pictures during different rotation frequencies from side views observing crystalline lens deformations under the influence of centrifugation.

A square function best represents the dependence of averaged and normalized flattening according to the rotational frequency, in order to compare the deformations with different kinds of cutting.

Flattening coefficients have turned out to be more and more important with rotation frequency: the crystalline lens diameter increased while its height decreased.

The tested crystalline lenses usually come back to their initial thickness (or thinnes) after the rotative test.

The crystalline lens flexibility obviously increases with the number of laser-cut sagittal planes: 8.2%, 16.6%, 26.6% for respectively 4, 8 and 12 sagittal planes (Fig. 4.16).

Gliding planes direction played a major part: the conical planes oriented in the emerging strength direction rose crystalline lens deformability.

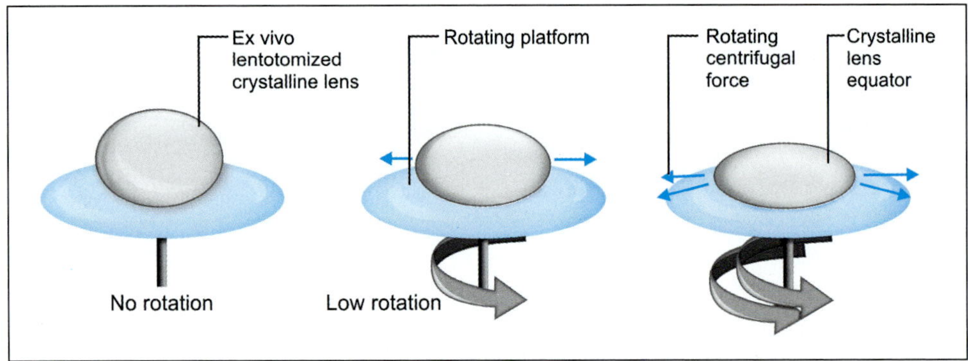

Fig. 4.17 Schematical representation of Fischer's apparatus, a device made to assess the effects of the rotating strength applied on ex vivo lentotomized crystalline lens

If crystalline lens capsule is both resistant and elastical enough, lentotomy should allow to retouch the whole crystalline lens, which would enable to reduce the accommodation loss.

4.3.1.2 Other Surgeries

Capsuloplasty is about laser treatment of the capsule with the aim of restoring deformability of the crystalline lens envelope.

Lens softening consists in using a low energy photodisruptive laser to improve the biomechanical characteristics of the lens nucleus.

Scientists dream is about having a phako-Ersatz (*See* paragraph 4.3.1, Phakomodulation, page 153) some day:

- from a punctiform aperture,
- empty bag filling, freed from its crystalline lens (Fig. 4.19), and
- with a solution available to refractive power adaptation under the effect of the tensional variations in the bag.

We will see later (*See* paragraph 4.4.3, Anteriorities, page 173) that this approach is under way, although lens capsules lose transparency during preservation process (Fig. 4.18).

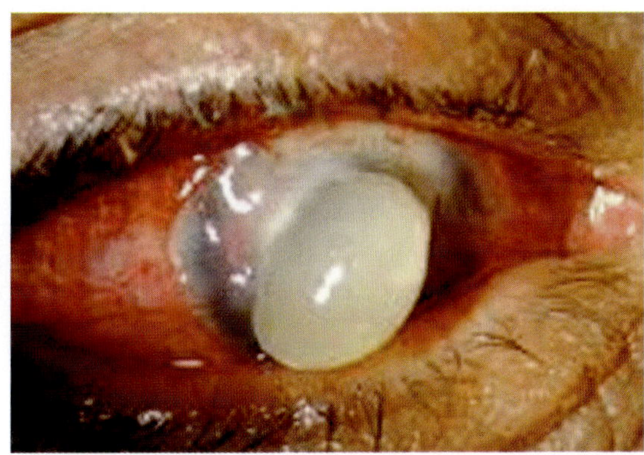

Fig. 4.18 Ex vivo human crystalline lens luxation in case of an ocular trauma

So tragic this picture may be for the patient, note that natural crystalline lens may lose its transparency as soon as dessicated, if outside the body fluids or damaged. Thus, ex vivo viscoelasticity properties of the crystalline lens may be changed for the experiments.

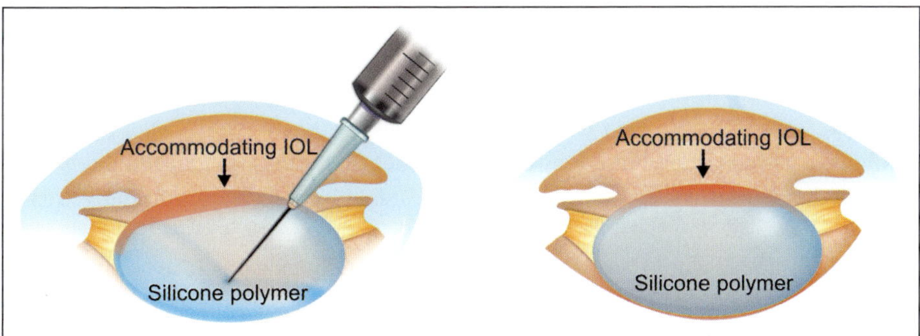

Fig. 4.19 Principles of phako-Ersatz

Phako-Ersatz may be concepted with (as shown on the scheme above) or without accommodating IOL in the capsular bag.

Hence, the present considerable stakes to control capsular opacification (*See also* paragraph 3.3.9.5, Surgical pearls with IOL, page 118) by means of different techniques:

- capsular polishing,
- distilled water, and
- antimitotics.

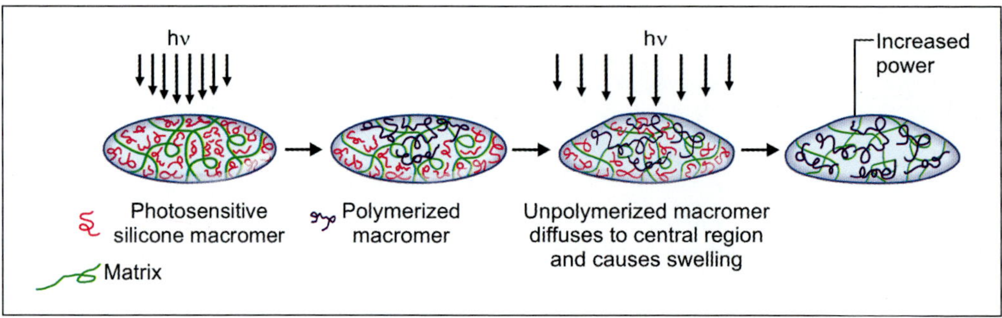

Fig. 4.20 Principles of LAL

The light adjustement of this IOL consists of a photopolymerization of the biomaterial constitutive of the implant. The beam laser is directed toward the center of the IOL to produce the physical process, then IOL is exposed to a final laser as a UV-blocker. This technique permits a fine tuning in IOL power to better control presbyopia as well.

There have been other attempts as for IOL adjustable to certain light wavelength, so-called light adjustable lens (LAL) (Fig. 4.20).

According to these various scleral and lenticular approaches, there is no identified technique offering a physiological, immediate and sustainable, stable and adjustable in time, accommodative restoration at the moment.

Associating the techniques would probably enable accommodative gain close to physiology.

To get these clinical results, it seems obvious to better evaluate the potential of the anatomical area, which is dramatically involved in accommodation: the ciliary zone (*See* Fig. 4.25).

4.3.2 Lentotomy

To treat presbyopia, Femtosecond (FS) laser-mediated incisions in crystalline lens body may be a therapeutical solution for some people (*See* paragraph 4.3.1.1, Femtosecond (FS) laser lentotomy, page 153).

FS lentotomy tests on living rabbit have been satisfactory, with no cataract induced, no retinal damage, nor adverse effects in ocular tissues 3 months after surgery.

In a series of experiments on human and porcine crystalline lenses, a German team has confirmed the increase of the crystalline lens flexibility using a 5 kHz or 100 kHz femtosecond laser with different cross-section profiles (*See* Fig. 4.16).

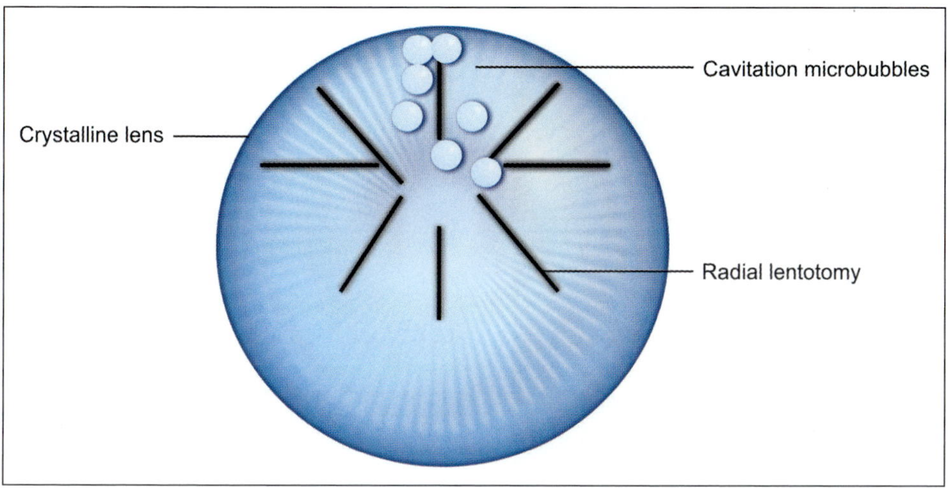

Fig. 4.21 Schematic image after wheel-radii shape lentotomy (from operating microscope view)

After lentotomy, the FS sculpture shape of 12-wheel-radii, respecting a 1-mm central free zone, in a radial surface, has given the best crystalline lens flexibility (Fig. 4.21).

With lentotomies, crystalline lens flexibility can increase up to 20%, although this percentage varies according to the crystalline lens age and state.

It is likely that incisions increase flexibility by behaving such as slip planes allowing the crystalline lens to deform under the action of pressure strength.

The restoration of the lenticular flexibility is supposed to allow the aging crystalline lens to accommodate again: 100 μm in human crystalline lens would restore up to 3 diopters of accommodative gain (*See also* paragraph 1.5.4, Accommodative structures, page 34).

Experiments on 15 rabbits have allowed to realize the microsurgical process in 25 seconds per eye, a factor 10 reduction as compared to the first attempts with lasers of lesser repetitive frequency.

The affordable duration of lentotomy makes the technique reliable to human.

OCT imaging and Scheimpflug of operated eyes had clearly showed the presence of bubbles and diffusion of light immediately after surgical procedure (Fig. 4.22).

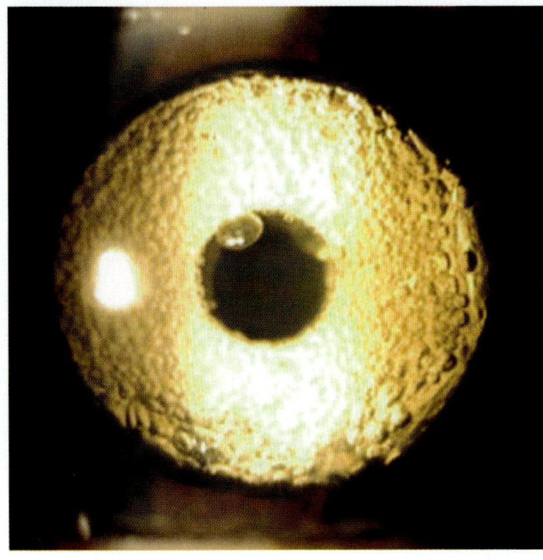

Fig. 4.22 Example of FS laser lentotomy in human for cataract extraction. Cavitation bubbles are well visible immediately after the procedure

Ultraspeed laser is also used on crystalline lens to perform modern cataract extraction without handpiece phako-emulsifier.

After 14 days, one and three months, the traces of incisions became blurred and the diffusion of light improved while microincisions healed up.

No kind of cataract was reported after 3 months and the lateral tissular damages remained localized.

Human can overcome the centering difficulty of the experimental treatment in rabbits by staring at a target.

The accurate setting of laser impacts, energy and spacing are of paramount importance for the evolution. Accurate measurements are necessary to insure the cutplanes distribution in the crystalline lens nucleus without crystalline capsule breaking.

The possible retinal damage remains an eventful complication, all the more since the laser pulses in the wavelength of close infrared are focused neerer to the retina than in the case of corneal lasers treatments.

Histological studies of treated eyes in rabbits showed no inflammatory sign nor degeneration.

4.3.3 Ciliary Exploration

In ophthalmology, to explore anterior segment, many imaging techniques are available (*See also* Figs 1.12, 1.13, 1.16. 2.1, 2.2 and 2.6).

4.3.3.1 Ciliary Imaging with OCT

Nonetheless, iris backward position (pigment mask) as well as small dimensions of ciliary ring and its revolution symmetry do not permit any study by explorations using neither:

- photonic energy [Scheimpflug images (*See also* Fig. 3.5)] nor,
- infrared light (optical coherence tomography or anterior segment OCT) (Fig. 4.23).

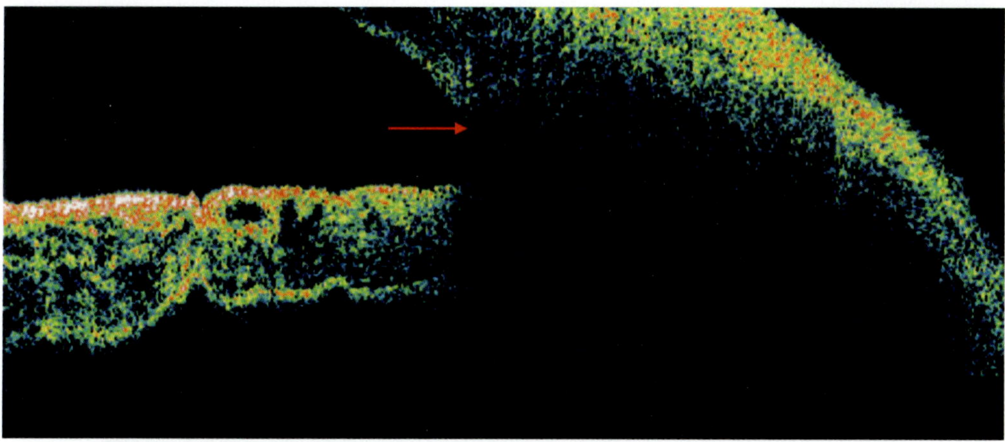

Fig. 4.23 OCT imaging of the iridocorneal angle (red arrow). Note that the signal is strongly attenuated by the sclera preventing analysis of this anatomical region (Personal iconography taken from a stratus OCT mounted with a 20 diopter additional lens)

The OCT technology mediated by the optical properties of the light is not indicated to explore the anatomical structures behind iris due to signal loss.

4.3.3.2 Ciliary Imaging with Scheimpflug

Scheimpflug photographical principle makes tridimensional exploration possible in light permeable tissues thanks to lateral beams coming from a frontal site of observation. This principle naturally goes with the exploration of ocular translucent zones (Fig. 4.24).

At this moment, only two medical devices allow a proper observation of the perilenticular zone: magnetic resonance imaging (MRI) or ultrasounds (US) technique (*See also* paragraph 1.5.3, Clinical approach, page 32).

Perilenticular space is the anatomical area around crystalline lens: zonule, ciliary zone, vitreous and aqueous humor (Fig. 4.25). Ciliary zone also has several anatomical distinct parts:
- Ciliary body:
    - Ciliary processes,
    - Ciliary muscle.
- Ciliary sulcus.

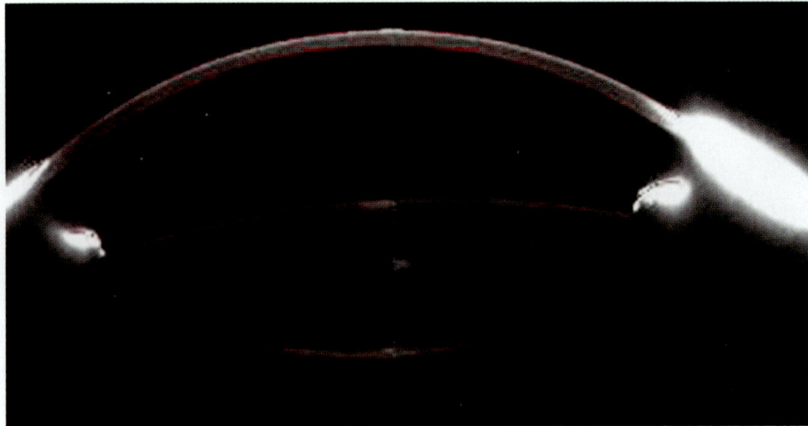

Fig. 4.24 Optical tomography of eye with Scheimpflug technique showing the anterior segment anatomy in front of iris (Personal iconography taken from an HD Okulus Pentacam)

High resolution (HR) technology in Scheimpflug camera allows accurate analysis of anterior segment without access to retroiris part.

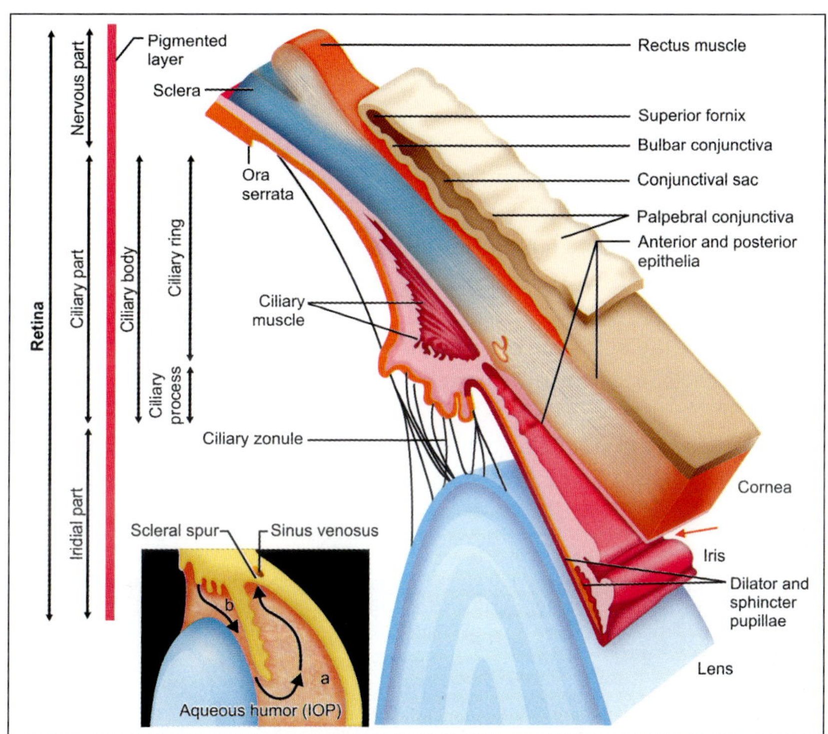

Fig. 4.25 Anatomy of the perilenticular space (red arrow) in the human

Perilenticular space is a not well-known anatomical part posterior to iris. This area is probably the clue of the accommodative process (a: anterior chamber and b: posterior chamber).

4.3.3.3 Ciliary Imaging with MRI

These techniques are:

- HR-MRI (still experimental level and developed by an American team from Piscataway) and,
- Artemis ultrasound apparatus, established by Dan Reinstein, Ron Silverman and Jackson Coleman.

Artemis uses a 50 MHz probe focused on cornea or anterior segment, but with arciform scanning so that it remains perpendicular to the cornea.

4.3.3.4 Ciliary Imaging with US

Thanks to US signal processing control, the accuracy of the measurements we have taken with apparatus is of 1 μm.

US was essential to know the anatomy of corneas operated on refractive surgery.

The device focusing on the anterior segment gave an image cut of complete anterior segment with a fair visualization of iridocorneal angle structures (Fig. 4.26).

US penetration of iris also enables to take sulcus-to-sulcus measurements for posterior chamber phakic implants, as we described it previously (*See also* paragraph 1.5.3, Clinical approach, page 32).

Today, US scanner represents the best source of images aimed at analyzing accommodative dynamics, with visualization of the ciliozonulolenticular modifications.

High resolution (HR) technique of MRI is not invasive and not optical, for it uses the properties of tissular atomic nuclei's magnetic resonance, static field, field gradients and pulsed radiofrequencies (Fig. 4.27).

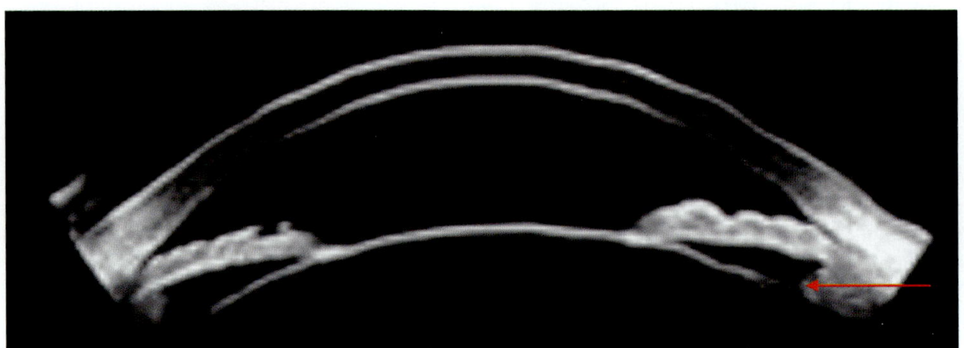

Fig. 4.26 Artemis US scanner imaging of anterior segment

Perilenticular space and posterior chamber (red arrow) are individualized with US technology cause, there is no decreasing in signal strength behind iris.

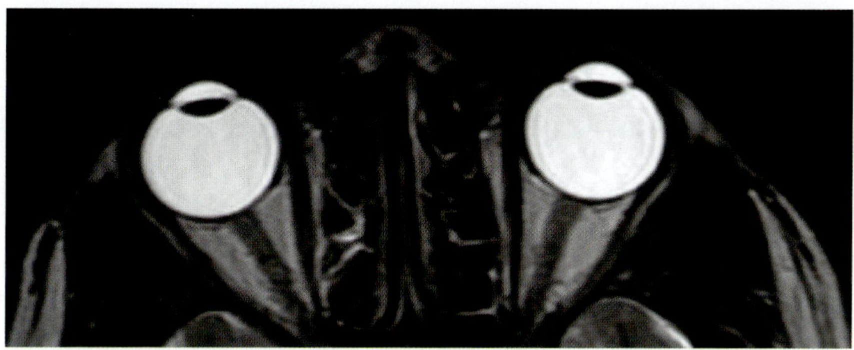

Fig. 4.27 Conventional MRI of the human eye (coronal view)

MRI allows to make analysis of different part of the body, especially anatomical structures rich in hydrogen atoms (such as liquids). Conventional MRI is limited because of the poor amplification of the images as in the case of eyeballs. HR-MRI increases dramatically the accuracy of the images obtained.

4.3.3.5 Results after Ciliary Exploration

MRI are free of distortion and optical reflection.

Moreover, this technique provides us with the advantage of unmatched contrast at the level of soft tissues, which represents intrinsic properties.

Contrast may vary according to the settings of pulse sequence radiofrequency time parameters.

We could catch pictures in all the planes of space desired.

HR-MRI, which the American team have developed for anterior segment imaging during accommodation, provides us with a visualization of ciliary muscle and of its geometrical links with crystalline lens (phakic subject), the optics or the implant haptics of IOL (pseudophakic subject).

Furthermore, HR-MRI does not interfere with vision while testing it. It then is worth testing binocular physiological accommodation, without the pharmacological induction of over accommodation (*See also paragraph 1.3.2, Miosis, page 13*).

At experimental level, and with a view to obtain HR pictures, MRI reaches 1.5 Tesla magnetic field.

HR-MRI gets a focuser especially dedicated to eye and uses a pulsed sequence radiofrequency, standard spin echo, balanced in T1, single echo and multicut.

Non-magnetic device was used to stimulate accommodation by watching pictures with disparity sent in the imager. Visual targets were at appropriate distance from eye to produce a strong binocular accommodative stimulus (until 8 diopters) or minimum (around 0.1 diopter) during the capture of MRI.

The distant target was presented through a mirror to exceed imager depth limits. During measurements, head stayed still and light was low.

Examined subjects were invited to watch the distant target: a black cross on a white background retroilluminated with optical fiber. Light intensity varied between 50% and 100%, at a pace of 2 alternative pictures a second. An initial series of measurements in orthogonal location was shot simultaneously in three dimensions, so that we could make out interest zone in 78 µm final resolution, 3-millimeter thick multicuts, on a field of 4 cm.

Target was repositioned to stimulate near vision before new images appear. The best contrast for ciliary muscle and ciliary processes differentiation was selected: ciliary processes were observed with a stronger signal intensity than the ciliary muscle, and lens cortex was lighter than the rest of the crystalline lens.

In posterior chamber pseudophakes, whether with monofocal or multifocal soft implants, accommodation came together with the appearance of a HR-MRI gap between ciliary processes and capsular bag equator, a space not observed in 80% of unaccommodated patients.

Measure equipment have also shown how crystalline lens sugery was connected with a deepening of the anterior chamber and of sulcus diameter increase.

In pseudophakes, accommodation came with a statistically significant reduction in:
- sulcus-to-sulcus distance,
- ciliary ring diameter,
- sulcus diameter, and
- irido-ciliary angle.

Capsular bag diameter containing the soft implant seemed to shrink significantly during accommodation.

If we then took the soft implant off the capsular bag, a circumlenticular space appeared again in most of the studied subjects.

A biometrical evaluation confirmed quasi-coincidence between capsular and ciliary planes:
- in 80% of implanted eyes,

- 20% having a posteriorized capsular plane compared with ciliary processes apex: they did not usually show the ordinary reduction of anterior chamber depth during accommodation, which we observed in pseudophakies (30 µm anterior chamber flattening).

The measurement of distance modifications between perpendicular to scleral spur and the ciliary sulcus showed great decrease in sulcus diameter during accommodation.

HR-MRI, which New Jersey Robert Wood Johnson University Hospital have developed, enables the visualization on the living:

- iris,
- ciliary muscle,
- ciliary processes, and
- crystalline lens.

And the measurement of the anatomical relations between these structures (no iris pigment obstruction).

HR-MRI offers the best contrast in soft tissues, useful for tissular (Fig. 4.27).

While we applied this imaging technique to anterior segment, we might use it to get information about:

- IOL position,
- behavior and study of accommodative mechanisms and presbyopic development.

HR-MRI study in presbyopic subjects has confirmed the changes in anterior segment structures associated with accommodation, and particularly important, it has proven that ciliary muscle contraction activity does not decline with aging but indeed seems to be maintained all life long.

Pictures obtained with HR-MRI confirm Helmholtz's theory (*See also* paragraph 1.5, Accommodative etiopathogenesis, page 28), at least regarding the increase with aging in crystalline lens thickness that the appearance of presbyopia involves.

Human uveal tractus reacts unambiguously as answer to the lenticular volume rise.

Although the lens performance usually decreases with aging, the modification in the ciliary muscle ring diameter during accommodation does not fall with aging (661 µm diameter variation, whatever the age of studied subjects).

This consequently excludes the notion of a certain atrophy degree coming with aging, despite usually taken it for granted to explain presbyopia.

In phakic subjects, ciliary muscle ring diameter depends on age for minimal and maximal accommodation:

It dramatically decreases with aging regardless the accommodative state (around 20 µm/year out of 20 years of presbyopia, meaning 400 µm between 40 and 60 years old).

In pseudophake, the reduction of ciliary muscle ring diameter and the loss in potential zonular tension following it, are compensated thanks to:

- IOL lesser volume (compared to naturel lens) associated with,
- capsular contraction with concomitant inward moving.

During accommodative efforts, and since the ciliary muscle efforts apparently influence the optic position, anteroposterior movements of IOL optic indicate that a certain level of zonular tension has come back after implantation (hence, the use of accommodative IOLs) (*See* paragraph 4.2.2, Accommodative IOLs, page 146).

HR-MRI may visualize IOL optics and haptics, and their relationship with anatomical structures involved in accommodation.

Accordingly, scleral therapeutical strategies would be likely to:

- increase the ciliary muscle ring diameter in presbyopic phakes and then,
- allow rise in circumlenticular space and then,
- imply increase in both zonular tension and accommodative answer (according to Helmholtz's theory so long as crystalline lens remains soft).

However, the lens continuous growth and effect on uveal tractus could reduce zonular tension and all potential accommodative answer.

Crystalline lens softening or filling surgical strategies (*See* paragraph 4.3.1, Phakomodulation, page 153), which do not reduce the lenticular volume or its equatorial diameter, should not be likely to:

- raise the circumlenticular space or,
- restore efficient tension in the zonule.

Considering that the contraction of the ciliary muscle did not decrease with aging or after IOL implantation in the capsular bag and considering that ciliary muscle diameter shrinks with aging (with or without implantation), we could modify the presbyopia correction strategy: taking into account functional ciliary muscle and ciliary muscle ring diameter, repercussion on zonular tension.

HR-MRI obtained anatomical and physiological consensus over a number of intraocular structures involved with accommodation.

Then, it seemed that:
- crystalline lens anterior surface described a paraboloid-shaped curve and that,
- during accommodation, the lens anteriorly translated but the posterior capsule stayed unchanged.

Presbyopic crystalline lenses:
- increased in volume and,
- flattened the anterior curvature.

There was some changes in:
- ciliary body and,
- only a part of Müller muscle that moved during accommodation.
  On the contrary, sulcus remained stable. It anatomically described an ellipsoidal-shaped ring, not circle.
  Posteriorly, zonule separated from ciliary processes to be a zonular contingent, said to be of secondary importance and, connected with the anterior vitreous: it is then entirely a part of the accommodative process.
  The presence of vitreous supports at the level of the lens confirms that there is a diaphragmatical mechanism, according to Coleman theory (*See also* paragraph 1.5.1, History, page 28).
  A Japanese team have suggested some accommodative restorations, in capsular bag and after lens standard phakoemulsification, by setting:
- two narrow implants in *piggy-back* before (*See also* paragraph 3.3.9.3, IOLs Piggy-backing, page 113),
- one injection, in the capsular bag and between both implants, of a biocompatible siliconed liquid with optical properties (optical indexes) and mechanical properties (viscoelasticity) (*See* Fig. 4.19): this enabled a certain degree of residual accommodation on double implant.
  As a result, presbyopia and accommodative restoration are better and better known thanks to the different studies using HR-MRI imaging techniques.

Today, accommodative restoration seems the most promising presbyopia method for emmetropes to improve their near vision without losing their distal vision. Ametropic patients can benefit from accommodative restoration after emmetropization by refractive surgery.

4.3.4 Ciliary Muscle Electrotransfer

At the moment, the development of the ocular systems for medication delivery is a booming research in ophthalmology (Fig. 4.28).

Electrotransfer potential applications could conceive a chemical approach to solve the problem of presbyopia: it is the most efficient nonviral technique in molecule delivery and we did not use it only for gene transfers.

Electrotransfer is an electrochemical technique that enables the polarized molecules to migrate through the ocular wall in electroinduced magnetic field.

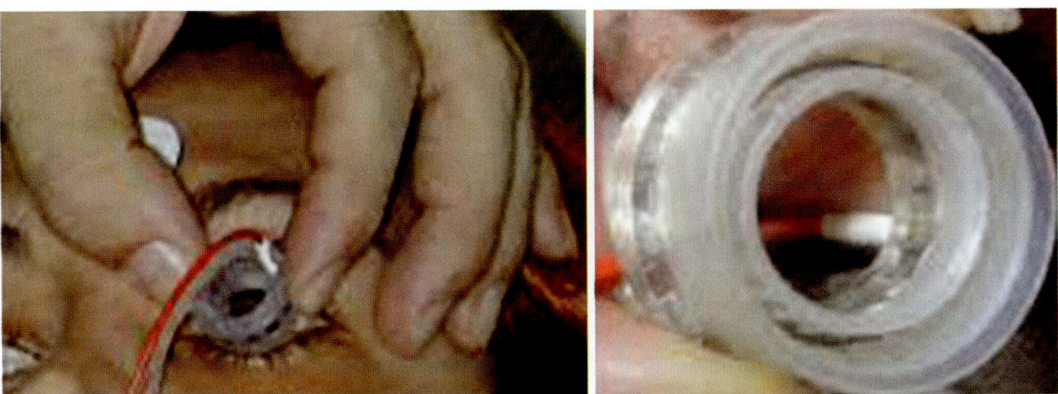

Fig. 4.28 Experiments of ocular electrotransferring in ciliary muscle

The principle of electrotransferring consists to place suction ring on the ocular surface (A). The ring of electrotransfer is mounted with a cathode (−) in the middle circle and an anode (+) connected to the periocular space by a patch. In the center of device, solution to be electrotransferred is poured, then the continuous current is switched on for the entire procedure.

Ciliary muscle might be used as a tank for intraocular expression and secretion of longtime therapeutic molecules.

Plasmid electrotransfer in ciliary muscle leads to the expression of reporting genes in the muscle fibers of the ciliary muscle during at least six months, according to a study in rats. Electrotransfer has been tested with plasmid bearing coding gene for human soluble receptors TNF-alpha.

Today, the plasmid electrotransfer in the ciliary muscle has neither induced any ocular illness nor any damage in ocular structure.

The production of heat shock proteins are chaperones molecules secreted by cells under different stresses. They have a protective function helping cells to cope with lethal conditions inducing apoptosis and cell differentiation. They maybe involved in tissue regeneration and may play a major role in presbyopia. Ciliary muscle happens to be useful to slow down the muscle degenerative process caused by presbyopia: we could proceed with a plasmid electrotransfer in order to produce the therapeutic proteins efficiently.

Besides, a possible muscular rejuvenation by muscle stimulation under the influence of growth hormone was to be considered.

A local hormone secretion by a ciliary muscle stimulated by a coding plasmid electrotransfer for this protein is feasible.

Thus, the electrotransfection of plasmids in the ciliary muscle as well as possibility to use the system of ciliary muscle proteins synthesis to produce proteins for a long time, gave us therapeutic perspectives (*See* Fig. 4.40).

4.3.5 Techniques of Lenticular Refilling

The final goal of cataract operation, beyond farsightedness restoration, is accommodative restoration.

The crystalline bag filling with an injectable polymer has potential to restore accommodation after cataract surgery (*See* Fig. 4.19).

However, two main difficulties have previously moderated the success of lenticular filling strategies.

First, the injected content leaked out of the capsular bag, then a secondary cataract appeared because of the loss of elasticity and the opacification of the capsular bag-crystalline lens anatomical complex.

Recently, we have developed lenticular filling simplified and highly reproducible processes with potential clinical applications to restore accommodation.

4.4 ACCOMMODATIVE EXPERIMENTAL SURGERY

As a matter of fact, since accommodation restoration seemed to be the best way to overcome this affection, we have joined the research and the development of an original surgical technique. It is all about carrying out what we could call "eye lifting".

It is not useless to remind that the device we present is under experimental and clinical evaluation and that, for now, does not prejudge the long-term functional result in presbyope.

4.4.1 Stakes

The history of ciliary distension ring development started with a preliminary project feasibility study that served as a prelude for potential partners.

Presbyopia is foreseeable and affects around 60% of French population, 100 million Europeans and more than 2 billion individuals thoughout the world. It represents the "holy Graal" of refractive surgery that we still have to control, an associated myopia, hyperopia and astigmatism correction, as we saw it in the previous chapters (*See also* chapter 3, Presbyopia and optical compensations, page 79). Better understanding of accommodative phenomenon should propose a corrective treatment for presbyopia via accommodation restoration rather than compensating surgery techniques:

- presbyLASIK (*See also* paragraph 3.3.7, PresbyLASIK, page 103),
- pseudo-accommodative IOLs (*See also* paragraph 3.3.9, Lenticular surgeries, page 109),
- conductive keratoplasty (*See also* paragraph 3.3.10, Conductive keratoplasty (CK), page 122).

Rather than various accommodative restoration attempts such as:

- anterior ciliary sclerotomy (*See* paragraph 4.1, Presbyopia and accommodative relaxation surgeries, page 137),
- scleral expansion bands (*See* paragraph 4.2.1, scleral expansion bands (SEBs), page 142).

Such as innovative techniques:

- Ciliozonular tension ring (CZTR),
- presbyring.

These techniques have showed real efficiency, the effect unfortunately facing regression within few weeks or months.

4.4.2 Concept

The original conception of the CZTR, personal patented device, would customize for each patient, in order to permit a readjustment with the evolution of presbyopia. It will also play a part in the intraocular lens support and in therapeutical vector during later improvement (*See* Fig. 4.40).

CZTR is a microring that:

- is implantable in presbyopic eye,
- under operating microscope,
- may be filled in central lumen that maintains it at its place and provides it with the effect of ciliary sulcus circumferential distension and anterior zonule by internal way (ciliozonular tension ring –CZTR– or zonulo-ciliary tension ring) (*See* paragraph 4.4.5, Patented invention of ciliozonular tension ring (CZTR), page 179).

From prototype conception to realization, there must be a meeting between the industrial partners who, via their research and development service, should validate concept and specifications, define the technological choices of the implantable material and the inflating CZTR.[6]

4.4.3 Anteriorities

With the intention of sharing new concept interest, in the official documents, we recapped our present knowledge of accommodation theories.

We also reminded that:

- According to Helmholtz, presbyopia stems from lens sclerosis added with capsule loss of elasticity, however, these signs lack at the beginning of presbyopia.
- According to Schachar, ciliary muscle continuous growth would lead to relaxation in the zonules tension, then preventing ciliary muscle from sufficiently modifying the shape of the lens.

In invention anteriorities research, we took into account the different techniques for accommodative restoration:

- Thornton invented the anterior ciliary sclerotomy (ACS) in the United States, in 1996 (Figs 4.29A and B),
- Fukasaku proposed the Japanese intrascleral implants in 1999 (Figs 4.29A and B),
- Schachar developed scleral prosthesis called scleral expansion bands (SEBs) (*See* paragraph 4.2.1, Scleral expansion bands (SEBs), page 142), for presbyopia treatment and other ocular troubles, then supraciliary segments (Baïkoff).

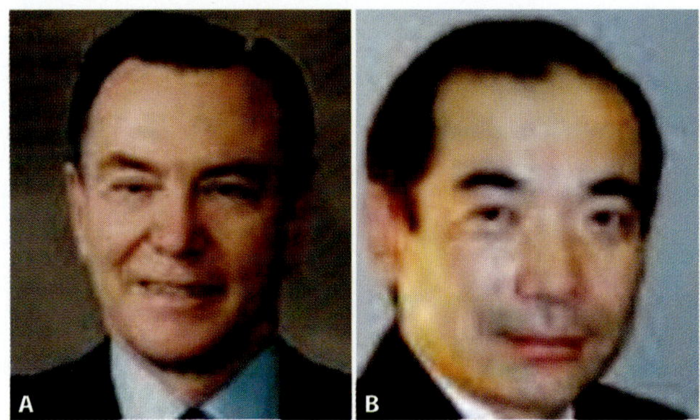

Figs 4.29A and B   First experiments of accommodative restoration by Thornton (A) with ACS, modified by Fukasaku (B) My own concept of accommodative restoration has to be compared with the pre-existing scleral techniques developed by predecessors.

The anterior ciliary sclerotomy, as we saw it previously *(See* paragraph 4.1.1, Blade anterior ciliary sclerotomy (ACS), page 138) consitsts of 8 radial incisions:

- in paralimbal sclera,
- being 2/3 deep or at 90% thickness (depending on authors).

Average increase in accommodative amplitude is of around 2 diopters but with the regression of effect in 6 months.

To avoid it, the improvement of the technique has been about making deeper incisions (100% of the thickness) and inserting a polydimethylsiloxane implant that suture keeps at the bottom of the incision. (*See* paragraph 4.1.2, ACS implant, page 139).

We also mentioned the various crystalline lens techniques dating back from 2004:

- according to dutch Koopman new injectable silicone to fill the lens up or,
- with a capsular plug after silicone intracapsular filling, according to Japanese Nishi's procedure (Fig. 4.30).

Koopman and Nishi proposed to restore accommodation in presbyopic patients having cataract by injecting, in the aperture made for prior cataract extraction, some fluid silicone in the capsular bag.

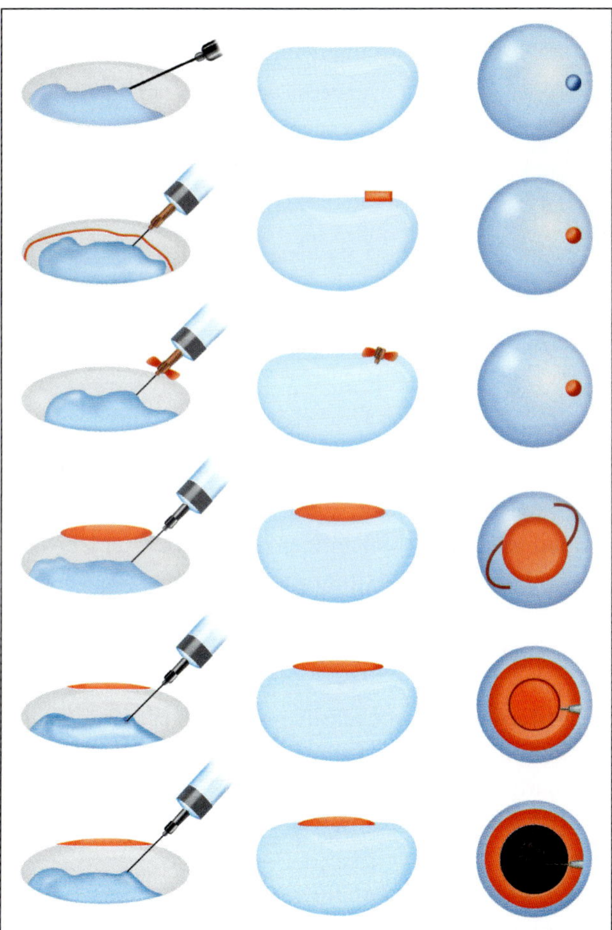

Fig. 4.30 First experiments of crystalline lens refilling with or without a capsular plug (3 upper schemes) to prevent liquid extrusion, with optional IOL in the bag (3 lower schemes)

My own concept of accommodative restoration has also to be compared with the pre-existing capsular techniques developed by predecessors.

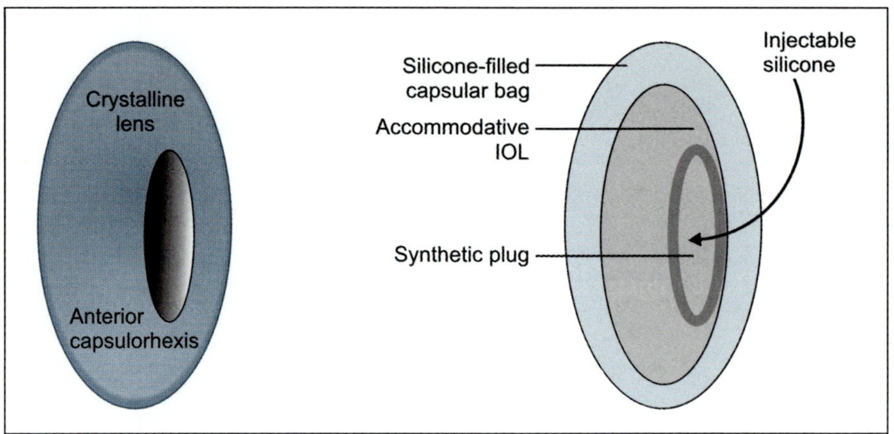

Fig. 4.31 Phako-Ersatz, lens plug and injected silicone, in accordance with Dr Nishi invention

AMO corporation developed two types of silicone: thanks to Glasser's device (*See also* paragraph 1.5.4, Accommodative structures, page 34), we plot postmortem animal measures between 4 and 8 accommodation diopters.

In monkeys, except for few complications, such as capsular fibrosis and postoperative inflammation, the experiments turned favorable.

Dr Nishi suggested the use of a plug to avoid all silicone leakages the anterior chamber (Fig. 4.30).

As a phako-Ersatz (*See* paragraph 4.3, Other surgeries of accommodation, page 153), he proposed to put in a lens 1.2 mm thick with a 13 mm diameter (Fig. 4.31).

Light adjustable material should allow to modify the anterior lens refractive power and adjust the accommodation (*See* Fig. 4.20).

Closer to our concept of CZTR reported other patented publications:

- French Ganem presbyring of 2003 (patent n° 98 16723, 31st, December 1998) following zonular tension ring published in 2002, during the Munich Congress Poster Session,
- The American Shahinpoor accommodating zonular minibridge implants, in 2003 (US 2003:0028248 A1) (Figs 4.32A and B).

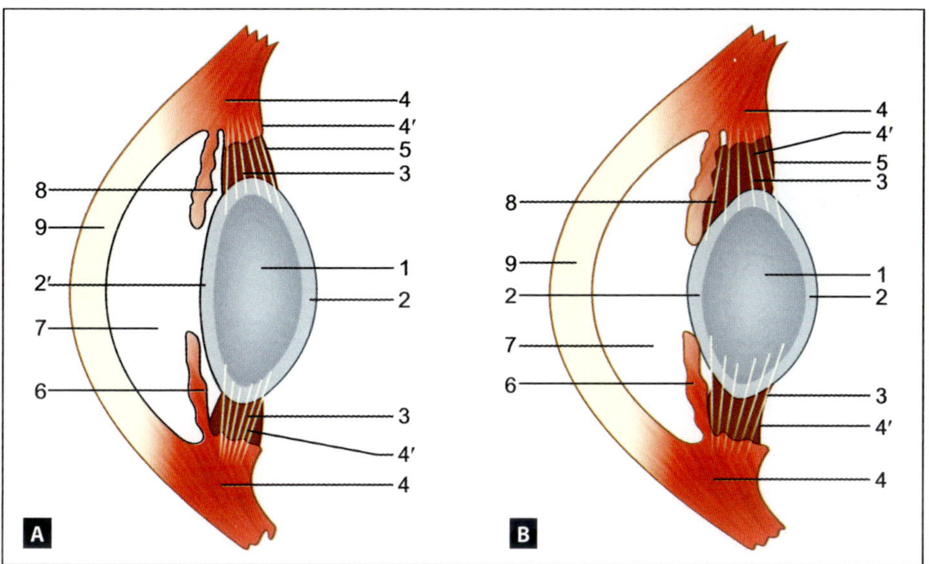

Figs 4.32A and B Shahinpoor zonular mini-bridge (legend 5) in place at rest (A) and during accommodation (B)

My own concept of accommodative restoration has also to be compared with pre-existing other zonular techniques developed by predecessors. Shahinpoor does not consider ciliary muscle defect, but aims to act directly on and in the zonule effector

4.4.4 Patent Claims

Ciliary zonular tension ring (CZTR) is distinct from Schachar device (US 6,280,468 B1:Scleral prosthesis for treatment of presbyopia and other eye disorders, 2001) on some points (*See* Fig. 4.41):

- scleral effect is related to an ab interno implantation,
- it settles in the ciliary sulcus and rests on the zonule (*See* Fig. 4.40).

Anteriority study puts forward an invention patent of a device that is circular, adjustable by liquid filling and implantable in cornea.

In 1999, Lee developed this implant to be implanted in cornea, the US under number 5.876.439 (Method and apparatus for adjusting corneal curvature using a fluid-filled corneal ring) (Figs 4.33 and 4.34).

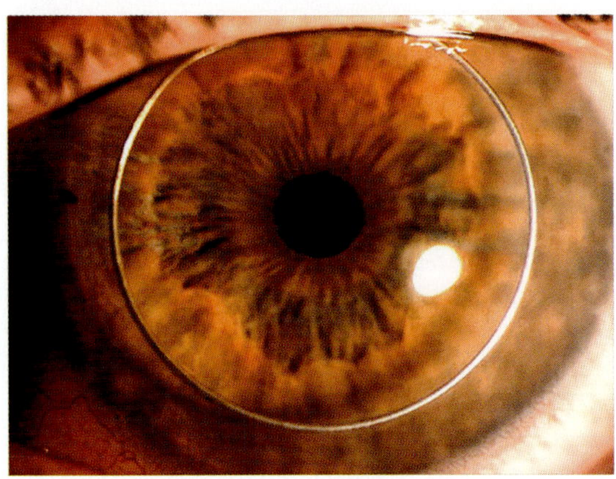

Fig. 4.33 Filled corneal ring according to Lee

My own concept of accommodative restoration has also to be compared with the pre-existing other corneal techniques developed by predecessors, even if far from an invention for correcting presbyopia.

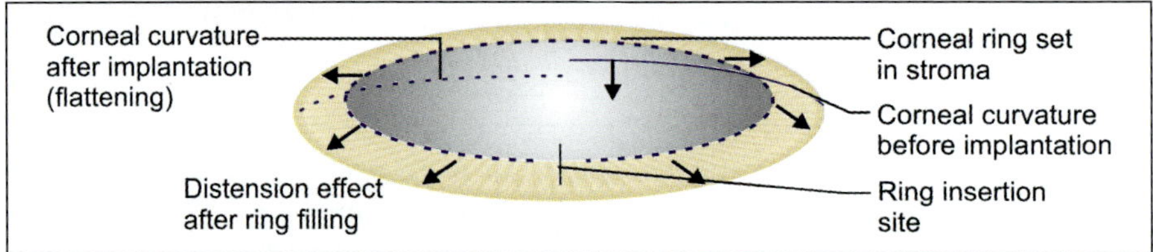

Fig. 4.34 Dr Lee fluid filling adjusting corneal ring

CZTR is clearly distinct from Lee's device since implantation must be in the cornea and not in the sulcus, despite similarities; indeed, both are circular devices with fluid filling (Fig. 4.34).

The same goes for the crystalline lens capsular tension ring during cataract surgery (Foldable Dick capsular ring type 2, Morcher Gmbh), a device that has nothing in common with our invention but its circular shape (*See also* Fig. 3.19).

Even closer to our invention, regarding conception and aim, is the French patent recorded as number 98 16723 (IOLTECH). It is about a device to treat presbyopia or other ocular affections: not adjustable device in hard (PMMA, polyHEMA) or soft (hydrogel) material (Fig. 4.35).

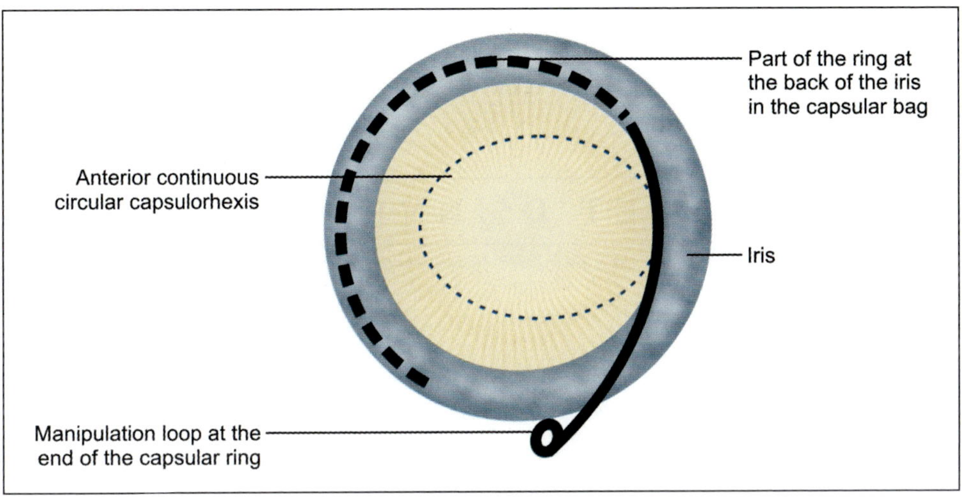

Fig. 4.35 Partially inserted capsular ring in the capsular bag.
The manipulation loop is clearly visible at the extremity of ring (Fig. 4.37)

Another French patent under number 99 08048 correcting presbyopia with an intraocular tension ring is distinct from our device as for:

- twisted shapes (slightly circular spring effect), and
- unadjustable (biocompatible material having enough shape memory to exert a spring effect).

4.4.5 Patented Invention of Ciliozonular Tension Ring (CZTR) (Fig. 4.36)

Our patent number FR0211870 consists in ciliozonular tension ring (CZTR):

- the shape of a ring,
- with aperture inferior to 100°,
- with a section diameter not exceeding 200 µm, and
- having a lumen accessible with micropunction or Duckbill microvalve or any other (Fig. 4.38).

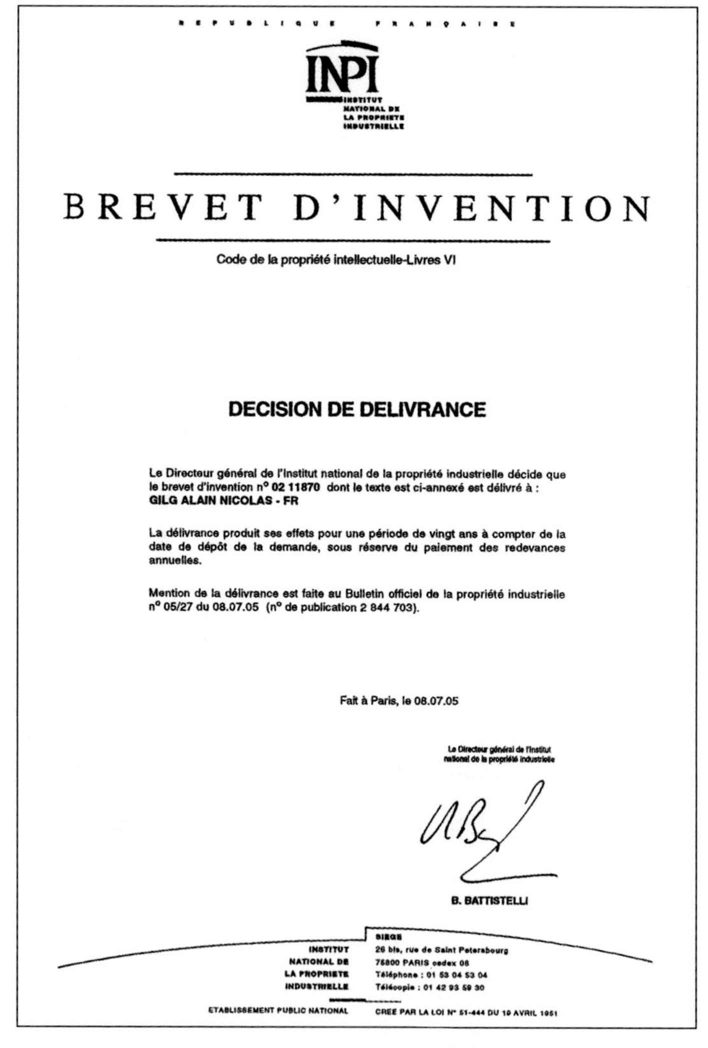

RÉPUBLIQUE FRANÇAISE

INPI

INSTITUT
NATIONAL DE
LA PROPRIÉTÉ
INDUSTRIELLE

BREVET D'INVENTION

Code de la propriété intellectuelle-Livres VI

DECISION DE DELIVRANCE

Le Directeur général de l'Institut national de la propriété industrielle décide que le brevet d'invention n° 02 11870 dont le texte est ci-annexé est délivré à :
GILG ALAIN NICOLAS - FR

La délivrance produit ses effets pour une période de vingt ans à compter de la date de dépôt de la demande, sous réserve du paiement des redevances annuelles.

Mention de la délivrance est faite au Bulletin officiel de la propriété industrielle n° 05/27 du 08.07.05 (n° de publication 2 844 703).

Fait à Paris, le 08.07.05

Le Directeur général de l'Institut
national de la propriété industrielle

B. BATTISTELLI

INSTITUT	SIEGE
NATIONAL DE	26 bis, rue de Saint Petersbourg
LA PROPRIETE	75800 PARIS cedex 08
INDUSTRIELLE	Téléphone : 01 53 04 53 04
	Télécopie : 01 42 93 59 30

ETABLISSEMENT PUBLIC NATIONAL   CREE PAR LA LOI N° 51-444 DU 19 AVRIL 1951

Fig. 4.36 Patented invention of CZTR (Fig. 4.38)

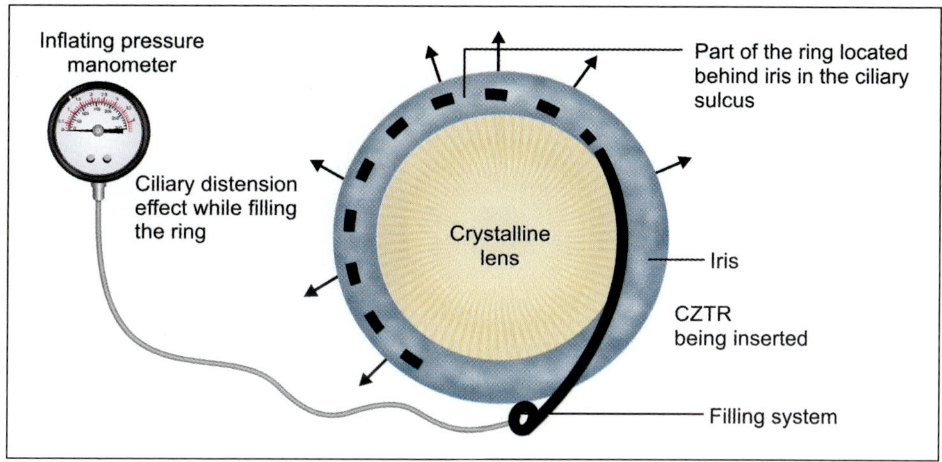

Fig. 4.37 Schematical patented CZTR prior to final position in ciliary sulcus. Pressure adjustment is being exerting sufficient counter-pressure in the sulcus (Fig. 4.35)

Inflatable system enables pressure and secondary ring distension control while inflating: beveled self-packing valves, by whistle-type catheter or free flap.

The CZTR material (Fig. 4.38):
- is biocompatible,
- soft,
- extensible,
- elastical,
- not porous,
- allows a lumen filling with fluid or gas, what then make distension of the external face of the device and permits to exert a tension against ciliary sulcus gutter and against the adjacent anterior fibers of the zonule (ellipsoid shape) (*See* paragraph 4.3.3, Ciliary exploration, page 161).
Valve process is made to adjust the pressure inside device, that is, to say to control pressure against the faces.

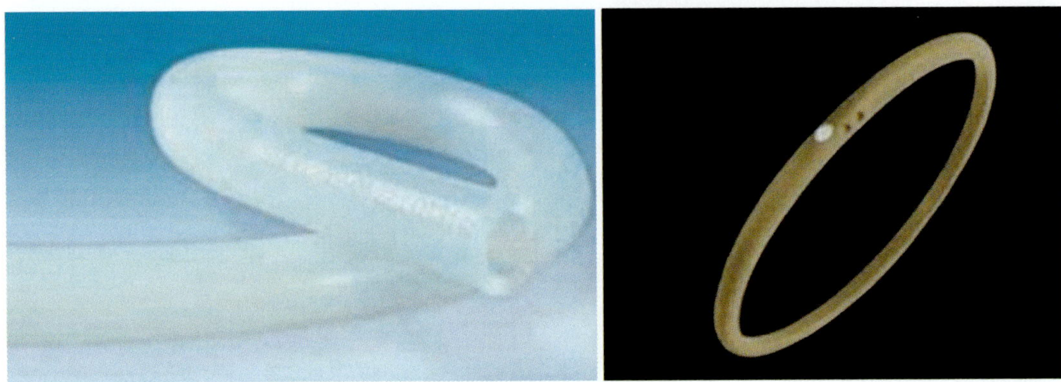

Fig. 4.38 Soft silicone microtubes to be used for experimental CZTR
CZTR must be soft to take exactly place in the ellipsoid sulcus gutter in humans

We fill the device with a micromanometer until obtaining the desired pressure for optimal efficiency, taking into account the anatomical dimensions of eye and the extent of presbyopia.

We implant the device into the eye:
- through a 2.2-mm corneal microincision, in the presence of viscoelastical substance,
- behind the iris, we then progressively inflate, and
- put it into ciliary sulcus.

Envelop has the shape of a ring or of a ring portion, with a external diameter predetermined at rest. Internal face delimits a lumen to be filled with incompressible fluid that tends to increase external diameter.

It rises up to a value for which we obtain a compensation of tension loss in zonular fibers.

If CZTR was made of hard material, then we could not insert it inside the eye after folding: the insertion of hard ring would require a wider corneal incision and potentially traumatic intraocular handling.

CZTR owns geometry that we predetermine while making it.

With predetermined diameter, CZTR gets invariable intrinsic spring effect, which avoids the possibility of several rings (sulcus diameter is around 11.2 mm and less then 2 mm wide).

CZTR must be able to exert distensive strength giving way to scleral ring dilation of 400 μm (crystalline lens diameter increasing of 400 μm with presbyopia, or 20 μm/year between 40 and 60 years old (*See* paragraph 4.3.3, Ciliary exploration, page 161).

The ring, whether open (between 1 and 100°) or closed (uniform contact over all the sulcus), should be able to adapt to each ciliary sulcus diameter and to all presbyopia levels (Fig. 4.38):
- external diameter measuring at rest between 10 and 11.5 mm, and inflated, between 12 and 13 mm,
- for 2 mm diameter and 200 μm thick envelop, lumen volume at rest is of 58 mm^3 to reach a bit more than 94 mm^3 (face thickness decrease neglected under stretching effect).

One size fits all: one unique size for the device suits all the implanted eyes (Fig. 4.38).

Annular tube must not exceed 2 mm after inflating (sulcus diameter) and envelop thickness is between 50 and 1000 μm (preference for lower values).

Lumen is filled with poor compressible biocompatible fluid or gas that allows to exert efficient pressure on the faces of the envelop (physiological saline solution).

CZTR is considered as being at rest when lumen is totally filled, without causing envelop dilation (micromanometer test) (Fig. 4.37).

Once introduced, the folded CZTR in eye is submitted to progressive and controlled unfolding during filling up.

We could control the position with ocular bioendomicroscopy[6] (under development) and the device could be repositioned or removed via the same corneal incision.

For the correction of spheric ametropias that are associated with presbyopia, CZTR also has bounds permitting concomitant or subsequent fixation of a phakic IOL (Fig. 4.39).

The gutter delimited by CZTR interior circumference serves as a support for precrystalline (phakic IOL) or pseudocrystalline (IOL) lens optic system (*See also* paragraph 3.3.9, Lenticular surgeries, page 109).

We could envisage different materials and include them in specifications:
- silicone (Fig. 4.38),
- polyolefin homopolymers or copolymers,
- urethane-based polyurethane or elastomers (polyurethane/methacryloyloxyethyl),

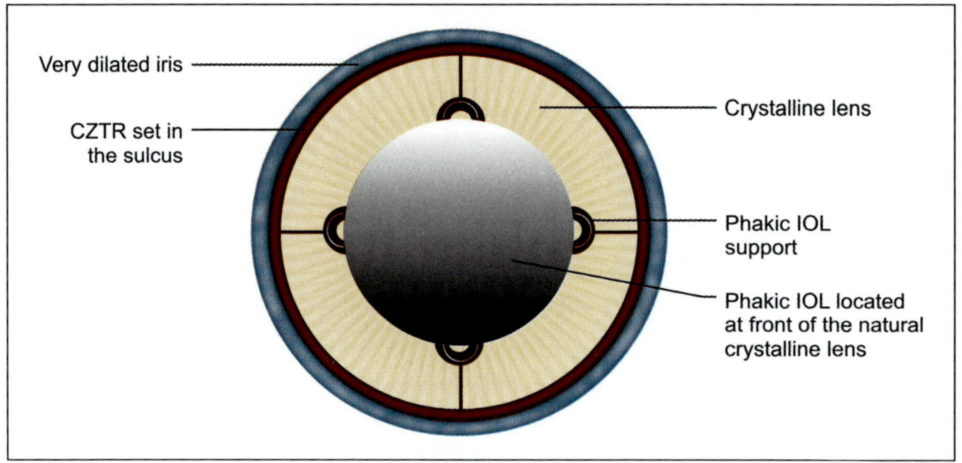

Fig. 4.39 From a front view, schematical CZTR set in the sulcus, with precrystalline phakic IOL optic

- polyacrylic,
- hydrogel, silico-hydrogel (organopolysyloxanes and polydiméthylsiloxanes), silicone-urethane,
- polycarbonate-urethane, polyether-etherketone, N-acyliminoethylene,
- bovine-hydrogel collagen,
- polyvinyl chloride elastomer (polyesters),
- polyethylene terephthalate, polytetrafluoroethylene, polymethyl methacrylate plastic, polysulphone, polyphosphazene,
- phosphorylcholine,
- silicone, natural rubbers (latex) or synthetic rubbers (butadiene and acrylic thermoplastic, butylstyrene, fluoropolyurethane, nylon, SIS/SBS elastomers, dexplastomers),
- alkylammonium-montmorillonite,
- Hytrel-type block copolymer, and
- dihydroxydiethyl ether and polytetramethylene dimethyl terephtalate, with a molecular weight between 600 and 3000 kDa.

Hytrel thus has got hard segments (4GT) and soft amorphous elastomer segments of polyalkylene terephthalate ether.

The judicious proportion of both components implies final product characteristics as far as solidity, elasticity, melting point, chemical resistance and permeability are concerned.

Active principle (steroids in the intermediate uveitis for instance, antiglaucoma agents, anticataract) could take place after envelop impregnation or setting of a prolonged-release system (Fig. 4.40).

By elastomer material, we mean a material that we can repeatedly stretch out, up to twice initial size, at physiological temperature, and which comes back to initial length after canceling stretching mechanical constraint:

- elastomers: ASTM F1441-92 and F2051-00 norm,
- thermoplastic elastomers: ASTM D5538-98 norm,
- silicone elastomers: ASTM F2038 and 2042 -00e1 norm (Fig. 4.38),
- olefine elastomer: ASTM D5593-99 e1 norm.

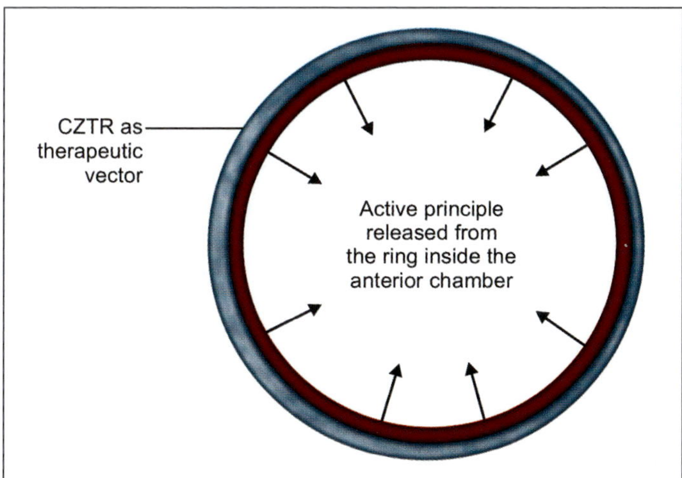

Fig. 4.40 Schematic CZTR set in the sulcus with a therapeutic vector function (Fig. 4.28)

With the experience of these specifications, CZTR was up for a feasibility assessment so as to show properties.

4.4.6 Feasibility Study

PTR n° 06.10.180 VRT commitment, from OSEO/ANVAR innovation and research services, has allowed to validate the feasibility study of such a device by proposing technical and technological developments:

- intelligent fluid material permitting to consider changing reversible solid/liquid state, then making device extraction and replacement possible by freeing from the valve,
- replacement of the liquid by a microscopic granular body available to be injected such as liquid and to avoid all long-term leakage necessitating implant replacement,
- in situ polymerization in order to adjust diameter, that is to say the pushing pressure against the sulcus.

Later research and development for improvement should call upon latest technologies as for microtechnique and nanotechnology to reach all required functionalities:

- hollow plastic ring that is,
- radially cracked,
- closed at ends, interior lumen previously filled via a leakage-tight microvalve with incompressible body with shape memory.

For the different types of ciliary rings (*See* paragraph 4.4.3, Anteriorities, page 173) that we presented earlier:

- Ganem's presbyring,
- IOLTECH's tension ring,
- experimental data confirm operative feasibility, good immediate clinic tolerance and above all favorable effect of accommodation restoration.

Patented CZTR (Fig. 4.41) is a microdevice, implantable in the ciliary sulcus in order to induce "scleral ring-lift", increasing circumlenticular space, which is the optimization of zonular fibers working distance. Original concept takes advantage to increase implant volume adapted to crystalline lens growth (*See* paragraph 4.3.3.5, Results after ciliary exploration, page 165). Continuous growth leads to inevitable loss in efficiency of devices proposed at the moment. We could obtain such volume variation by "inflating" during nanotechnological maintenance process.

In animal experiment presbyring ring slightly moves the zonules backward, without damaging it.

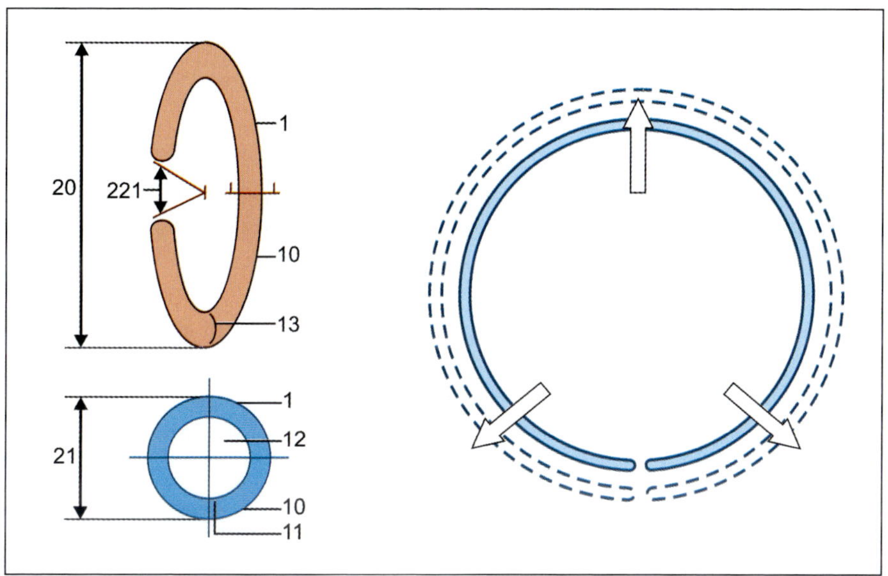

Fig. 4.41 Adjustable CZTR as described in Gilg's patent

In implanted Yucatan mini pigs (accommodative dimensions and behavior similar to humans), we did not notice hypertonia after 3 months, neither intraocular inflammation nor crystalline lens transparency impairment.

Accommodation amplitudes ranged from 3.5 to 4 diopters.

According to others, the device implanted in sulcus would have the effect to push back zonular fibers released in presbyopic eyes.

Out of 5 implanted pig eyes, CZTR has increased the pharmacological accommodation between 2 and 3.5 diopters, without microscopic lesion.

The zonular fibers stretching by CZTR is effectively supposed to rise the accommodative power.

In humans, CZTR are being evaluated.

These results would explain themselves regarding how the drop in accommodation amplitude is mainly due to loss in zonular fibers tension (*See* Fig. 4.1):
- crystalline lens diameter increase,
- loss of efficiency in vitreous humor movements (*See also* Fig. 1.14),
- olefin elastomer.

During accommodation, the circular ciliary muscle moves towards crystalline lens, the anterior radial ciliary muscle moves towards sclera and the consequences of both muscles combined action are:
- equatorial zonule stretching by the first contingent of collagen fibers,
- posterior zonule relaxation,
- ciliary processes move towards crystalline lens by the second contingent of collagen fibers.

Equatorial zonule passes on the anterior radial ciliary muscle, which entails rise in crystalline lens equatorial diameter.

Posterior and anterior zonules keep crystalline lens at place during accommodation (*See also* paragraph 1.5.1, History, page 28).

During ciliary contraction, through the radial and longitudinal ciliary muscles, there are simultaneously:
- equatorial zonule stretching and,
- anterior and posterior zonules relaxation (Fig. 4.42).

The presence of collagen fibers, between the anterior part of the radial muscle/ciliary sulcus and between ciliary muscle/ciliary processes, prove that the accommodation comes with both:
- equatorial zonule stretching and
- posterior fibers relaxation.

With aging, the continuous growth of crystalline lens associated with non-growing sclera, involves decrease in ciliary muscle working distance, and then loss of stretching capacity in zonular fibers.

Thus, studied CZTR is able to be applied against ciliary sulcus, if we want the equatorial zonular anchorage to move, in order to trigger the stretching again.

Surgery of CZTR can come with the other scleral expansion methods [sclerotomy (*See* paragraph 4.1, Presbyopia and accommodative relaxation surgeries, page 137), bands (*See* paragraph 4.2, Presbyopia and implant accommodative surgeries, page 142)].

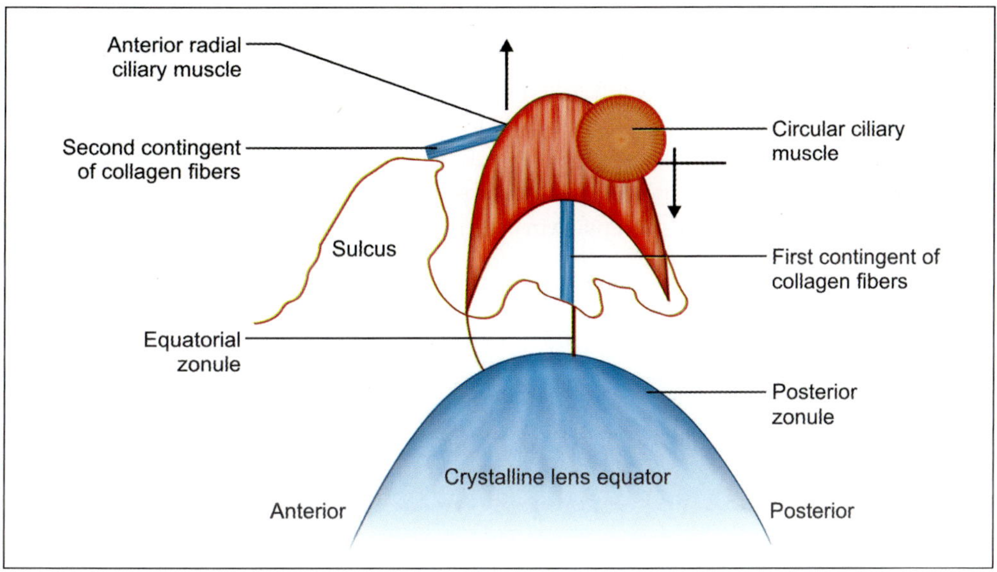

Fig. 4.42 Schematic profile view of ciliary movements during accommodation

Once in the sulcus and filled up, CZTR ensures a surface tension that spreads over the sulcus modifying:

- ciliary body distance with,
- arching in the peripheral anterior vitreous,
- stretching of the zonular fibers that become active again for efficient accommodation.

IOP concomitantly decreases due to uveoscleral trabecular improvement.

For ophthalmologists, scientists and patients, thanks to the improvement of the scleral techniques (*See* paragraph 4.1, Presbyopia and accommodative relaxation surgeries, page 137) and the promising future of lenticular techniques (*See* paragraph 4.3.5, Techniques of lenticular refilling, page 171), accommodative restoration as a presbyopia treatment is impending reality.

Experimental clinical results will be here to prove it, but the number of scientific publications remains too low to appreciate the extent.

The lack of predictibility with these techniques hampers their diffusion amongst our patients for now.

However, developing phako-Ersatz by replacement of the natural crystalline lens with an artificial lens presenting the same opticophysical properties, we would still have to face the inescapable decrease of circumlenticular space with aging. This decrease would be resolved by scleral techniques to increase zonular (*See* paragraph 4.3.3.5, Results after ciliary exploration, page 165) working distance and make phako-Ersatz functional again (*See* paragraph 4.1, Presbyopia and accommodative relaxation surgeries, page 137).

Then, if we improve our understanding of accommodative physiology, all these techniques are complementary and will naturally find their place in the future therapeutic arsenal of our operating theaters.

No others medical specialities than ophthalmology has none benefited from extraordinary progress years past. We are in the middle of this tremendous period when new ideas and major discoveries for our field abound.

Refractive surgery, a subspecialty in ophthalmology field, has recently taken off and kepts improving dramatically; since this surgery now concerns mainly all the spherocylindrical ametropias (myopias, hyperopias, astigmatisms). It also concerns selective aberropias, high order aberrations related visual troubles.

All these visual impairments can be taken and treated separately in young subjects who are not presbyope yet. However, in presbyopic, we also have to compensate or treat presbyopia, despite the risk of an increasing difficulty to intermediate vision, followed with a deterioration of nearsightedness.

As for presbyopic concomitant treatment, complexity lies in the misknowledge of intimate phenomena, prelude to presbyopia settling, which have firstly incited ophthalmologists to compensate presbyopia as a static ametropia.

These approximations have led some authors to develop compensating surgical techniques that remain imperfect because of the slow outcome of presbyopia with time and of therapeutical side effects on visual quality.

Other writers have thus searched for dynamical solutions to presbyopia so as to imitate accommodative physiology. Since we do not know thoroughly accommodative physiology, scleral and lenticular techniques have effects limited, in both amplitude and time. Here we are on the cutting edge between ocular tissues and the wound healing that we can hardly influence.

What about to treat presbyopia today? We will certainly be up for it in a very close future, whereas first clinical results for scleral and lenticular techniques are already very satisfactory.

We would be proud if we could, thanks to these reflexions, enrich the knowledge in the field of presbyopia treatment and inform the other visual health professionals about the actual state of presbyopia and its treatments[7].

We cheerfully invite our enthusiastic colleagues, friends and patients to actively participate to the setting up of a real therapeutic outline for the permanent treatment of presbyopia.

Still some time to go and myth will come true.

Notes

[Note 1]

I want to thank my supervisor, Professor Yves Pouliquen, then Ophthalmology Department Service Chief of the Hôtel-Dieu in Paris. While I was working by his sides, in the INSERM unity attached to his service, he showed me the way, during my postgraduate in biomaterials, he showed me the importance of the rigor while analyzing experimental facts and their clinical application. His work, a book called *The eye's transparency* (*La Transparence de l'oeil*), published in 1992 by Odile Jacob editors, relates with talent and poetry the whole epic story of the vision. He there talks about presbyopia in the "Aging eye" chapter with alterations of the crystalline lens, the vitreous body and the retina.

[Note 2]

I recommend André Vergez' work "Diagnosis in ophthalmology" (*Diagnostic en ophtalmologie*), published in Diffusion Générale de Librairie, Maloine, which is a sort of encyclopedic ophthalmological Vade-mecum in French, pocket size over 725 pages, unique of its kind regarding the amount of clinical knowledge methodically gathered in this book. The writer, a medical school teacher and hospitals ophthalmologist, died in 1978, just before his two works were released : the *Volume I, Eye and General Pathology* lists all the affections that can interfere with ophthalmology, the *Volume II*, identifies all the ocular affections from the symptoms. This book results from a huge work.

[Note 3]

In optometric terminology, progressive lenses for presbyopia may be sorted out in two groups. The group of visionaute characterized by people wearing spectacles with wide eye movement to alternate far and near vision. The group of spationaute who takes special care to move their neck and head to look around.

[Note 4]

In Ophtalmo review number 1, himself and his colleague, ENT specialist, propose a recent update on the sensorio-proprioceptive postural deficiency syndrome called "The sensorio-proprioceptive postural deficiency syndrome or ophthalmology differently" (Gilg AN, Aillagon-Bourguet L, April-May 2007, pp. 4-8). There is recalled the definition, the clinic and handling of the dysproprioception. This syndrome, which many European teams have recently discovered, is the subject of a thorough study about its relations with dyspraxia, dyslexia and the chronical and atypical pains in grown-ups. The treatment can be whether the wearing of postural reprogrammation soles, wearing prism presbyopic glasses (active prismation), bite-guard wearing, orthopractical re-education, vestibular re-education.

[Note 5]

Q in the central 20° to an average of 0.13 in the myopic presby-LASIKs against 0.50 in the witness group.

[Note 6]

Biomicroendoscopy is a surgical technique of intraocular imaging by means of soft microendoscope introduced though corneal incision, to observe and manipulate in anterior and posterior chamber of the eye under topical anesthesia. Gilg AN, Leon C, Leon J, Aron Rosa D, Klein RJ. Contribution of Ocular Endomicrosurgy in Presbyopia. A preliminary study of the accommodation in human. ESCRS, Sep 2001, Amsterdam.

[Note 7]

Many thanks to Caroline Kovarski who supported me, especially as far as the writing is concerned, she managed me and encouraged me to add diagrams and iconography in my text and helped a lot as for final reading of the book.

Bibliography

Articles

1. Investigating presbyopic options. Davis EA, Miller M, McDonald MB, Lindstrom RL, Yilmaz OF, Koch PS. *EyeWorld.* 2009 May;14(5):48-9.

2. Multifocal intraocular "mix and match" lenses. Lacmanovic-Loncar V, Pavicic-Astalos J, Petric-Vickovic I, Mandie Z. *Acta Clin Croat.* 2008 Dec;47(4):217-20.

3. Interocular blur suppression and monovision. Collins MJ, Goode A. *Acta Ophthalmol* (Copenh). 1994 Jun;72(3):376-80.

4. New aspects of contact lenses in ophthalmology. Aquavella Jv. *Adv Ophthalmol.* 1976;32:2-34.

5. Flight-deck vision of professional pilots. Watkins RD. *Aerosp Med.* 1970 Mar;41(3):337-42.

6. Reduced visual acuity in elderly people: the role of ergonomics and gerontechnology. Pinto MR, De Medici S, Zlotnicki A, Bianchi A, Van Sant C, Napoli C. *Age Ageing.* 1997 Sep;26(5):339-44.

7. Post-traumatic unilateral aphakia and contact lens-binocular functions of grown-ups. Ehrich W, Kolbegger K. Albrecht Von Graefes *Arch Klin Exp Ophthalmol.* 1975 Nov 25;197(2):177-92. German.

8. Femtosecond lasers in ophthalmology. Soong HK, Malta JB. *Am J Ophthalmol.* 2009 Feb;147(2):189-197. e2. Epub 2008 Oct 18. Review.

9. Maximizing satisfaction with presbyopia-correcting intraocular lenses: the missing links. Pepose JS. *Am J Ophthalmol.* 2008 Nov;146(5):641-8. Epub 2008 Sep 13. Review.

10. Presbyopia correcting intraocular lenses: what do I do? Olson RJ. *Am J Ophthalmol.* 2008 Apr;145(4):593-4.

11. The quality of life associated with presbyopia. Luo BP, Brown GC, Luo SC, Brown MM. *Am J Ophthalmol.* 2008 Apr; 145(4):618-622. Epub 2008 Feb 19.

12. New intraocular lens technology. Olson RJ, Werner L, Mamalis N, Cionni R. *Am J Ophthalmol.* 2005 Oct;140(4):709-16. Epub 2005 Jul 18. Review.

13. Implantation of scleral expansion band segments for the treatment of presbyopia. Qazi MA, Pepose JS, Shuster JJ. *Am J Ophthalmol.* 2002 Dec;134(6):808-15.

14. A complication of scleral expansion surgery for treatment of presbyopia. Singh G, Chalfin S. *Am J Ophthalmol.* 2000 Oct;130(4):521-3.

15. Correction of presbyopia accompanied by alternating exotropia. To'mey KF, Fahd SD, Jabbour NM. *Am J Ophthalmol.* 1982 Jul;94(1):125.

16. Aspherical deformation of lenses with variable refractive power. Zander K, Rassow B. *Am J Optom Arch Am Acad Optom.* 1972 Nov;49(11):938-42.

17. Some seeing problems: spectacles, color, driving and decline from age and poor lighting. Richards Ow. *Am J Optom Arch Am Acad Optom.* 1972 Jul;49(7):539-46.

18. Analysis of bifocal contact lenses. Wesley NK. *Am J Optom Arch Am Acad Optom.* 1971 Nov;48(11):926-31.

19. Presbyopia as a human factor in industry. Hill GC. *Am J Optom Arch Am Acad Optom.* 1971 Jul;48(7):556-9.

20. Stereopsis in presbyopes fitted with single vision contact lenses. Koetting RA. *Am J Optom Arch Am Acad Optom.* 1970 Jul;47(7):557-61.

21. Further data on presbyopia in different ethnic groups. Hofstetter HW. *Am J Optom Arch Am Acad Optom.* 1968 Aug;45(8):522-7.

22. The single vision reading contact lens. Fleischman WE. *Am J Optom Arch Am Acad Optom.* 1968 Jun;45(6):408-9.

23. Prescribing for presbyopia with contact lenses. Bier N. *Am J Optom Arch Am Acad Optom.* 1967 Nov;44(11):687-710.

24. Patterns of binocular suppression and accommodation in monovision. Schor C, Erickson P. *Am J Optom Physiol Opt.* 1988 Nov;65(11):853-61.

25. Stereopsis in presbyopes wearing monovision and simultaneous vision bifocal contact lenses. McGill E, Erickson P. *Am J Optom Physiol Opt.* 1988 Aug;65(8):619-26.

26. Comparative investigations of progressive lenses. Diepes H, Tameling A. *Am J Optom Physiol Opt.* 1988 Jul;65(7):571-9.

27. Monovision contact lens wear and occupational task performance. Sheedy JE, Harris MG, Busby L, Chan E, Koga I. *Am J Optom Physiol Opt.* 1988 Jan;65(1):14-8.

28. Ocular dominance and the interocular suppression of blur in monovision. Schor C, Landsman L, Erickson P. *Am J Optom Physiol Opt.* 1987 Oct;64(10):723-30.

29. Bifocal adds and environmental temperature. Kragha IK, Hofstetter HW. *Am J Optom Physiol Opt.* 1986 May;63(5):372-6.

30. A system of retinoscopy for the aged eye. Carter JH. *Am J Optom Physiol Opt.* 1986 Apr;63(4):298-9.

31. Suppression behavior analyzed as a function of monovision addition power. Heath DA, Hines C, Schwartz F. *Am J Optom Physiol Opt.* 1986 Mar;63(3):198-201.

32. Eye and head contribution to gaze at near through multifocals: the usable field of view. Afanador AJ, Aitsebaomo P, Gertsman DR. *Am J Optom Physiol Opt.* 1986 Mar;63(3):187-92.

33. Adaptation to lens-induced heterophorias. North R, Henson DB. *Am J Optom Physiol Opt.* 1985 Nov;62(11):774-80.

34. Performance characteristics of a hydrophilic concentric bifocal contact lens. Erickson P, Robboy M. *Am J Optom Physiol Opt.* 1985 Oct;62(10):702-8.

35. Clinical factors in proximal vergence. Wick B. *Am J Optom Physiol Opt.* 1985 Jan;62(1):1-18.

36. Depth of field for the presbyope. Carroll JP. *Am J Optom Physiol Opt.* 1981 May;58(5):400-3.

37. Spectacles for the emmetropic presbyopic optometrist. Goodlaw El. *Am J Optom Physiol Opt.* 1981 Mar;58(3):232-4.

38. Vision training for presbyopic nonstrabismic patients. Wick B. *Am J Optom Physiol Opt.* 1977 Apr;54(4):244-7.

39. The design and prescription of multifocal lenses for civil pilots. Backman HA, Smith FD. *Am J Optom Physiol Opt.* 1975 Sep;52(9):591-9.

40. Bifocal contact lenses today. Lahr JW. *Am J Optom Physiol Opt.* 1975 Aug;52(8):547-58.

41. Depth of focus and amplitude of accommodation through trifocal glasses. MILES pw. *AMA Arch Ophthalmol.* 1953 Mar;49(3):271-9.

42. Optogeometric considerations regarding corrective lenses used in ametropia and presbyopia. JUNES. *Ann Ocul* (Paris). 1953 Oct;186(10):918-42.

43. Cause and treatment of presbyopia with a method for increasing the amplitude of accommodation. Schachar RA. *Ann Ophthalmol.* 1992 Dec;24(12):445-7, 452.

44. Rapid refraction. Beasley FJ. *Ann Ophthalmol.* 1971 Aug; 3(8):827-8.

45. Anterior ciliary sclerotomy using collagen T-shaped implants for treatment of presbyopia. Malyugin B, Antonian S, Lohman BD. *Ann Ophthalmol* (Skokie). 2008 Fall-Winter, 40(3-4):130-6.

46. Presbyopia correction: managing the complex patient. Hardten DR. *Ann Ophthalmol* (Skokie). 2007 Jun;39(2): 92-4, 91.

47. Cataract surgery and spectacle independence. Packer M. *Ann Ophthalmol* (Skokie). 2007 Spring;39(1):3-8. Review.

48. Current viewpoints concerning contact lenses. Urvoy M, Elie G, Carre V, Toulemont PJ. *Année Ther Clin Ophthalmol*. 1988;39:93-102, discussion 141-53.

49. The choice of eyeglass lenses in modern life. Catros A, Mur J. *Année Ther Clin Ophthalmol*. 1986;37:49-58.

50. Multifocal eyeglasses: rules for prescription. Catros A, Carrica A, Botaka E. *Année Ther Clin Ophthalmol*. 1983;34:135-49.

51. Progressive lenses. Catros A. *Année Ther Clin Ophthalmol*. 1972;23:339-49.

52. Optical surface optimization for the correction of presbyopia. Dai GM. *Appl Opt*. 2006 Jun 10;45(17):4184-95.

53. Global vision impairment due to uncorrected presbyopia. Holden BA, Fricke TR, Ho SM, Wong R, Schlenther G, Cronjé S, Burnett A, Papas E, Naidoo KS, Frick KD. *Arch Ophthalmol*. 2008 Dec;126(12):1731-9.

54. Multifocal corneal topographic changes with excimer laser photorefractive keratectomy. Moreira H, Garbus JJ, Fasano A, Lee M, Clapham TN, McDonnell PJ. *Arch Ophthalmol*. 1992 Jul;110(7):994-9.

55. Presbyopia. Bito LZ. *Arch Ophthalmol*. 1988 Nov; 106(11):1526-7. *Aust NZ J Ophthalmol*. 1991 Aug; 19(3):243.

56. The correction of refractive errors without surgery. Milder B. *Aust N Z J Ophthalmol*. 1989 Aug;17(3):261-4.

57. Comparison of bifocal and progressive addition lenses on aviator target detection performance. Markovits AS, Reddix MD, O'Connell SR, Collyer PD. *Aviat Space Environ Med*. 1995 Apr;66(4):303-8.

58. Social skills training for depressed, visually impaired older adults. A treatment manual. Donohue B, Acierno R, Hersen M, Van Hasselt VB. *Behav Modif*. 1995 Oct;19(4):379-424.

59. Objective measurement of aniseikonia: initial clinical results. Gernet H. *Bibl Ophthalmol*. 1975;(83):294-300.

60. Uncorrected refractive error and presbyopia: accommodating the unmet need. Bourne RR. *Br J Ophthalmol*. 2007 Jul;91(7):848-50.

61. Refractive surgery. McDonnell PJ. *Br J Ophthalmol*. 1999 Nov; 83(11):1257-60. Review.

62. Ophthalmologic problems of the elderly. De Voe AG. *Bull NY Acad Med*. 1978 Jun;54(6):561-7.

63. How to correct presbyopia. Pereleux A. *Bull Soc Belge Ophthalmol*. 1997;264: 63-6.

64. Correction of presbyopia with soft multivision lenses. Coursaux G, Corbe C, Saraux H, Massin M. *Bull Soc Ophthalmol Fr*. 1989 Jun-Jul;89(6-7):831-3.

65. For the rehabilitation of the presbyopic patient, a new "progressive bifocal" lens. Manent PJ, Pecheur J, Maille M, Claude R. *Bull Soc Ophthalmol Fr*. 1980 Oct;80(10):851-6.

66. Objective assessment of aberrations induced by multifocal contact lenses in vivo. Patel S, Fakhry M, Alió JL. *CLAO J*. 2002 Oct;28(4):196-201.

67. Visual performance of a multi-zone bifocal and a progressive multifocal contact lens. Guillon M, Maissa C, Cooper P, Girard Claudon K, Poling TR. *CLAO J*. 2002 Apr;28(2):88-93.

68. An objective and subjective comparative analysis of diffractive and front surface aspheric contact lens designs used to correct presbyopia. Brenner MB. *CLAO J.* 1994 Jan;20(1):19-22.

69. Stereopsis in anisometropically fit presbyopic contact lens wearers. Kastl PR. *CLAO J.* 1983 Oct-Dec;9(4):322-3.

70. Restoration of accommodation: surgical options for correction of presbyopia. Glasser A. *Clin Exp Optom.* 2008 May;91(3):279-95.

71. New thinking about presbyopia. Atchison DA. *Clin Exp Optom.* 2008 May;91(3):205-6.

72. Comparison of diffractive and refractive multifocal intraocular lenses in presbyopia treatment. Barisić A, Dekaris I, Gabrić N, Bohac M, Romac I, Mravicić I, Lazić R. *Coll Antropol.* 2008 Oct;32 Suppl2: 27-31.

73. Theoretical basis for the scleral expansion band procedure for surgical reversal of presbyopia [SRP]. Schachar RA. *Compr Ther.* 2001 Spring;27(1):39-46.

74. Refractive lens exchange for presbyopia. Kashani S, Mearza AA, Claoué C. *Cant Lens Anterior Eye.* 2008 Jun;31(3):117- 21. Epub 2008 Apr 11. Review.

75. An exploration of modified monovision with diffractive bifocal contact lenses. Freeman MH, Charman WN. *Cont Lens Anterior Eye.* 2007 Jul;30(3):189-96. Epub 2007 Feb 7.

76. Treatment of presbyopia with conductive keratoplasty: six-month results of the 1-year United States FDA clinical trial. McDonald MB, Durrie D, Asbell P, Maloney R, Nichamin L. *Cornea.* 2004 Oct;23(7):661-8.

77. Aspheric intraocular lens selection: the evolution of refractive cataract surgery. Packer M, Fine IH, Hoffman RS. *Curr Opin Ophthalmol.* 2008 Jan;19(1):1-4.

78. Conductive keratoplasty. Du TT, Fan VC, Asbell PA. *Curr Opin Ophthalmol.* 2007 Jul;18(4):334-7. Review.

79. Accommodative intraocular lenses: considerations on use, function and design. Doane JF, Jackson RT. *Curr Opin Ophthalmol.* 2007 Jul;18(4):318-24. Review.

80. Phakic intraocular lenses. Chang DH, Davis EA. *Curr Opin Ophthalmol.* 2006 Feb;17(1):99-104. Review.

81. Surgical treatment of presbyopia: scleral, corneal, and lenticular. Baikoff G. *Curr Opin Ophthalmol.* 2004 Aug;15(4):365-9. Review.

82. Advances in phakic intraocular lenses: indications, efficacy, safety, and new designs. Alio JL. *Curr Opin Ophthalmol.* 2004 Aug;15(4):350-7. Review.

83. Accommodating intraocular lenses. Doane JF. *Curr Opin Ophthalmol.* 2004 Feb;15(1):16-21. Review.

84. Presbyopic contact lenses. Atwood JD. *Curr Opin Ophthalmol.* 2000 Aug;11(4):296-8. Review.

85. Refractive cataract surgery. Kershner RM. *Curr Opin Ophthalmol.* 1998 Feb;9(1):46-54. Review.

86. Refraction, including prisms. Hiatt RL. *Curr Opin Ophthalmol.* 1991 Feb;2(1):63-8. Review.

87. Accommodative dysfunction. Daum KM. *Doc Ophthalmol.* 1983 May 1;55(3):177-98.

88. Accommodation, convergence and aging. Breinin GM, Chin NB. *Doc Ophthalmol.* 1973 Feb 21;34(1):109-21.

89. Presbyopia: an animal model and experimental approaches for the study of the mechanism of accommodation and ocular ageing. Bito LZ, Kaufman PL, DeRousseau CJ, Koretz J. *Eye.* 1987;1(Pt 2):222-30. Review.

90. Contrast visual acuity with bifocal contact lenses. Ueda K, Inagaki Y. *Eye Contact Lens.* 2007 Mar;33(2):98-102.

91. Quality of vision with presbyopic contact lens correction: subjective and light sensitivity rating. Alongi S, Rolando M, Corallo G, Siniscalchi C, Monaco M, Sacca S, Verrastro G, Menoni S, Ravera GB,

Calabria G. *Graefes Arch Clin Exp Ophthalmol.* 2001 Sep;239(9):656-63.

92. Clearer vision: visual freedom through multifocal lenses. Polefka KC. *Insight.* 2006 Oct-Dec;31(4):15-7, quiz 18-9.

93. Good subjective presbyopic correction with newly designed aspheric multifocal contact lens. Zandvoort SW, Kok JH, Molenaar H. *Int Ophthalmol.* 1993-1994;17(6):305-11.

94. Scleral expansion procedure for the correction of presbyopia. Kleinmann G, Kim HJ, Yee RW. *Int Ophthalmol Clin.* 2006 Summer;46(3):1-12. Review.

95. Presbyopic surgery. Schachar RA. *Int Ophthalmol Clin.* 2002 Fall;42(4):107-18. Review.

96. Anterior ciliary sclerotomy with silicone expansion plug implantation: effect on presbyopia and intraocular pressure. Fukasaku H, Marron JA. *Int Ophthalmol Clin.* 2001 Spring;41(2):133-41. Review.

97. The surgical reversal of presbyopia: a new procedure to restore accommodation. Marmer RH. *Int Ophthalmol Clin.* 2001 Spring;41(2):123-32. Review.

98. Correction of presbyopia with the excimer laser. Epstein O, Vinciguerra P, Frueh BE. *Int Ophthalmol Clin.* 2001 Spring;41(2):103-11. Review.

99. Bifocal contact lenses in presbyopia. Van Meter WS, Hainsworth KM, Duff C, Litteral G. *Int Ophthalmol Clin.* 2001 Spring;41(2):71-90. Review.

100. The correction of presbyopia. Schachar RA. *Int Ophthalmol Clin.* 2001 Spring;41(2):53-70. Review.

101. Laser correction of hyperopia and presbyopia. Anschütz T. *Int Ophthalmol Clin.* 1994 Fall;34(4):107-37. Review.

102. The accommodation requirement in myopia and hyperopia. Contact lenses versus spectacles. Hermann JS. *Int Ophthalmol Clin.* 1971 Winter;11(4):217-24.

103. Explanation for good visual acuity in uncorrected residual hyperopia and presbyopia after radial keratotomy. Hemenger RP, Tomlinson A, McDonnell PJ. *Invest Ophthalmol Vis Sci.* 1990 Aug;31(8):1644-6.

104. What's new in ophthalmic surgery? Coleman DJ. *J Am Coll Surg.* 2003 Nov;197(5):802-5. Review.

105. Role of protein molecular and metabolic aberrations in aging, in the physiologic decline of the aged, and in age-associated diseases. Tollefsbol TO, Cohen HJ. *J Am Geriatr Soc.* 1986 Apr;34(4):282-94. Review.

106. Presbyopia. Copeland AM. *J Am Optom Assoc.* 1992 Jul;63(7):463-4.

107. The effect of monovision lenses on the nearpoint range of single binocular vision. McGill EC, Erickson P. *J Am Optom Assoc.* 1991 Nov;62(11):828-31.

108. Low vision aids and the presbyope. Dillehay SM, Pensyl CD. *J Am Optom Assoc.* 1991 Sep;62(9):704-10.

109. The Tangent Streak rigid gas permeable bifocal contact lens. Remba MJ. *J Am Optom Assoc.* 1988 Mar;59(3):212-6.

110. Potential range of clear vision in monovision. Erickson P. *J Am Optom Assoc.* 1988 Mar;59(3):203-5.

111. Monovision vs. aspheric bifocal contact lenses: a crossover study. Josephson JE, Caffery BE. *J Am Optom Assoc.* 1987 Aug;58(8):652-4.

112. A critical view of presbyopic add determination. Hanlon SO, Nakabayashi J, Shigezawa G. *J Am Optom Assoc.* 1987 Jun;58(6):468-72.

113. Photopic pupillometry-guided laser in situ keratomileusis for hyperopic presbyopia. Assil KK, Chang SH, Bhandarkar SG, Sturm JM, Christian WK. *J Cataract Refract Surg.* 2008 Feb;34(2):205-10.

114. First safety study of femtosecond laser photo-disruption in animal lenses: tissue morphology and cataractogenesis. Krueger RR, Kuszak J, Lubatschowski H,

Myers RI, Ripken T, Heisterkamp A. *J Cataract Refract Surg.* 2005 Dec;31(12):2386-94.

115. Anterior chamber inflammation induced by conductive keratoplasty. Moshirfar M, Feilmeier M, Kumar R. *J Cataract Refract Surg.* 2005 Aug;31(8):1676-7.

116. Additional payments for presbyopia-correcting intraocular lenses. Mamalis N. *J Cataract Refract Surg.* 2005 Aug;31(8):1467-8.

117. Multifocal IOLs for presbyopia. Versteeg FF. *J Cataract Refract Surg.* 2005 Jul;31(7):1266, author reply 1266.

118. Optical coherence tomography of scleral expansion band implantation. Schachar RA. *J Cataract Refract Surg.* 2005 Jan;31(1):12.

119. Near vision restoration with refractive lens exchange and pseudoaccommodating and multifocal refractive and diffractive intraocular lenses: comparative clinical study. Alió JL, Tavolato M, De la Hoz F, Claramonte P, Rodriguez-Prats JL, Galal A. *J Cataract Refract Surg.* 2004 Dec;30(12):2494-503.

120. Accommodating intraocular lenses. Mamalis N. *J Cataract Refract Surg.* 2004 Dec;30(12):2455-6.

121. Secondary procedures after presbyopic lens exchange. Leccisotti A. *J Cataract Refract Surg.* 2004 Jul;30(7):1461-5.

122. Correction of presbyopia with refractive multifocal phakic intraocular lenses. Baï koff G, Matach G, Fontaine A, Ferraz C, Spera C. *J Cataract Refract Surg.* 2004 Jul;30(7):1454-60.

123. Evaluation of a satisfied bilateral scleral expansion band patient. Ostrin LA, Kasthurirangan S, Glasser A. *J Cataract Refract Surg.* 2004 Jul;30(7):1445-53.

124. Imaging scleral expansion bands for presbyopia with optical coherence tomography. Wirbelauer C, Karandish A, Aurich H, Pham DT. *J Cataract Refract Surg.* 2003 Dec;29(12):2435-8.

125. Comparison of myopes and hyperopes after laser in situ keratomileusis monovision. Goldberg DB. *J Cataract Refract Surg.* 2003 Sep;29(9):1695-701.

126. Refractive lens exchange with the array multifocal intraocular lens. Packer M, Fine IH, Hoffman RS. *J Cataract Refract Surg.* 2002 Mar;28(3):421-4.

127. Laser in situ keratomileusis monovision. Goldberg DB. *J Cataract Refract Surg.* 2001 Sep;27(9):1449-55.

128. Binocular function and patient satisfaction after monovision induced by myopic photorefractive keratectomy. Wright KW, Guemes A, Kapadia MS, Wilson SE. *J Cataract Refract Surg.* 1999 Feb;25(2):177-82.

129. Small-diameter corneal inlay in presbyopic or pseudophakic patients. Keates RH, Martines E, Tennen DG, Reich C. *J Cataract Refract Surg.* 1995 Sep;21(5):519-21.

130. Refractive changes induced by electrocautery of the rabbit anterior lens capsule. Jungschaffer DA, Saber E, Zimmerman KM, McDonnell PJ, Feldon SE. *J Cataract Refract Surg.* 1994 Mar;20(2):132-7.

131. Pathophysiology of accommodation and presbyopia. Understanding the clinical implications. Schachar RA. *J Fla Med Assoc.* 1994 Apr;81(4):268-71. Review.

132. The new generation of diffractive multifocal intraocular lenses. Wang IJ, Hu FR. *J Formos Med Assoc.* 2009 Feb;108(2):83-6.

133. Presbyopia surgery: principles and current indications. Saragoussi JJ. *J Fr Ophthalmol.* 2007 May;30(5):552-8.

134. Comparison of high-order optical aberrations induced by different multifocal contact lens geometries. Peyre C, Fumery L, Gatinel D. *J Fr Ophthalmol.* 2005 Jun;28(6):599-604.

135. Multifocal phakic intraocular lens implant to correct presbyopia. Baikoff G, Matach G, Fontaine A, Ferraz C, Spera C. *J Fr Ophthalmol.* 2005 Mar;28(3):258-65.

136. Current concept and developments in restoration of accommodation after cataract surgery. Serdarevic O. *J Fr Ophthalmol.* 2003 Sep;26(7):662-4.

137. Anisometropia and presbyopia: prescription of progressive lenses, a new approach. Pouliquen de Liniere M, Hervault C, Meillon JP, Rocher P, Coulombel P, Van Effenterre G. *J Fr Ophthalmol.* 1998 May;21(5):321-7.

138. Study of spatial function using the contrast sensitivity function. Cases of presbyopic subjects fitted with progressive glasses. Monot A, Chiron A, Cottin F, Bourdy C. *J Fr Ophthalmol.* 1986;9(3):199-209.

139. Compensating presbyopia: a new physiological progressive lens. Manent PJ, Pecheur J, Maille M, Claude R. *J Fr Ophthalmol.* 1981;4(11):757-61.

140. Pseudoaccommodative cornea treatment using the NIDEK EC-5000 CXIII excimer laser in myopic and hyperopic presbyopes. Uy E, Go R. *J Refract Surg.* 2009 Jan;25(1 Suppl):S148-55.

141. LASIK for hyperopic astigmatism and presbyopia using micro-monovision with the Carl Zeiss Meditec MEL80 platform. Reinstein DZ, Couch DG, Archer TJ. *J Refract Surg.* 2009 Jan;25(1):37-58.

142. In vivo application and imaging of intralenticular femtosecond laser pulses for the restoration of accommodation. Schumacher S, Fromm M, Oberheide U, Gerten G, Wegener A, Lubatschowski H. *J Refract Surg.* 2008 Nov;24(9):991-5.

143. Application of the polychromatic defocus transfer function to multifocal lenses. Schwiegerling J, Choi J. *J Refract Surg.* 2008 Nov;24(9):965-9.

144. Introduction to the proceedings of the 9th International Congress of Wavefront and Presbyopic Refractive Corrections. Applegate RA, Krueger RR. *J Refract Surg.* 2008 Nov;24(9):963-4.

145. Multifocal corneal ablation for hyperopic presbyopes. Jung SW, Kim MJ, Park SH, Joo CK. *J Refract Surg.* 2008 Nov;24(9):903-10.

146. More on peripheral PresbyLASIK as a centerdistance technique. Pinelli R. *J Refract Surg.* 2008 Sep;24(7):665.

147. Is peripheral presbyLASIK a center-distance technique? de Ortueta D. *J Refract Surg.* 2008 Jun;24(6):561, author reply 562.

148. Correction of presbyopia in hyperopia with a center-distance, paracentral-near technique using the Technolas 2l7z platform. Pinelli R, Ortiz D, Simonetto A, Bacchi C, Sala E, Alió JL. *J Refract Surg.* 2008 May;24(5):494-500.

149. Pseudoaccommodation and visual acuity with Technovision presbyLASIK and a theoretical simulated Array multi focal intraocular lens. Illueca C, Alió JL, Mas D, Ortiz D, Perez J, Espinosa J, Esperanza S. *J Refract Surg.* 2008 Apr;24(4):344-9.

150. Comparison of Acri. Smart multifocal IOL, crystalens AT-45 accommodative IOL, and Technovision presbyLASIK for correcting presbyopia. Patel S, Alió JL, Feinbaum C. *J Refract Surg.* 2008 Mar;24(3):294-9.

151. Analysis of the optical performance of presbyopia treatments with the defocus transfer function. Schwiegerling J. *J Refract Surg.* 2007 Nov;23(9):965-71.

152. Conductive keratoplasty for presbyopia: 3-year results. Stahl JE. *J Refract Surg.* 2007 Nov;23(9):905-10.

153. An alternative method for dominant eye test. Wang X, Fu J, Zhao S. *J Refract Surg.* 2007 Jun;23(6):536, author reply 536.

154. Optical analysis of presbyLASIK treatment by a light propagation algorithm. Ortiz D, Alió JL, Illueca C, Mas D, Sala E, Pérez J, Espinosa J. *J Refract Surg.* 2007 Jan;23(1):39-44.

155. Prediction and control of corneal asphericity after refractive surgery. Lin JT. *J Refract Surg.* 2006 Nov;22(9):848-9.

156. Bifocal profiles and strategies of presbyLASIK for pseudoaccommodation. Lin JT. *J Refract Surg.* 2006 Oct;22(8):736-8.

157. Correction of presbyopia by technovision central multifocal LASIK (presbyLASIK). Alió JL, Chaubard JJ, Caliz A, Sala E, Patel S. *J Refract Surg.* 2006 May;22(5):453-60.

158. Conductive keratoplasty for presbyopia: l-year results. Stahl JE. *J Refract Surg.* 2006 Feb;22(2):137-44.

159. Update of presbyopia treatment by scleral ablation using Er: YAG and UV lasers. Lin JT, Kadambi V. *J Refract Surg.* 2006 Jan-Feb;22(1):16-7, author reply 17.

160. Objective quality of vision in presbyopic and non-presbyopic patients after pseudoaccommodative advanced surface ablation. Cantú R, Rosales MA, Tepichin E, Curioca A, Montes Y, Ramirez-Zavaleta JG. *J Refract Surg.* 2005 Sep-Oct;21(5 Suppl):S603-5.

161. Monovision LASIK for pre-presbyopic and presbyopic patients. Cheng AC, Lam DS. *J Refract Surg.* 2005 Jul-Aug;21(4):411-2, author reply 412.

162. Monovision LASIK for pre-presbyopic and presbyopic patients. Goldberg DB. *J Refract Surg.* 2005 Jul-Aug;21(4):411, author reply 412.

163. Ocular integrity after anterior ciliary sclerotomy and scleral ablation by the Er: YAG laser. Ito M, Asano-Kato N, Fukagawa K, Arai H, Toda I, Tsubota K. *J Refract Surg.* 2005 Jan-Feb;21(1):77-81.

164. Ablation design in relation to spatial frequency, depth-of-focus, and age. Charman WN. *J Refract Surg.* 2004 Sep-Oct;20(5):S542-9. Review.

165. Pseudo-accommodative cornea: a new concept for correction of presbyopia. Telandro A. *J Refract Surg.* 2004 Sep-Oct;20(5 Suppl):S714-7.

166. Advanced surface ablation for presbyopia using the Nidek EC-5000 laser. Cantú R, Rosales MA, Tepichin E, Curioca A, Montes Y, Bonilla J. *J Refract Surg.* 2004 Sep-Oct;20(5 Suppl):S711-3.

167. Monovision laser in situ keratomileusis for pre-presbyopic and presbyopic patients. Miranda D, Krueger RR. *J Refract Surg.* 2004 Jul-Aug;20(4):325-8.

168. Diode laser thermal keratoplasty to correct hyperopia. Rehany U, Landa E. *J Refract Surg.* 2004 Jan-Feb;20(1):53-61.

169. Treatment of presbyopia by infrared laser radial sclerectomy. Lin JT, Mallo O. *J Refract Surg.* 2003 Jul-Aug;19(4):465-7.

170. An informal satisfaction survey of 200 patients after laser in situ keratomileusis. Hill JC. *J Refract Surg.* 2002 Jul-Aug;18(4):454-9.

171. Scleral expansion surgery does not restore accommodation in human presbyopia. Elander R. *J Refract Surg;*1999 Sep-Oct;15(5):604.

172. Centered vs. inferior off-center ablation to correct hyperopia and presbyopia. Bauerberg JM. *J Refract Surg.* 1999 Jan-Feb;15(1):66-9.

173. Lens thickness with age and accommodation by optical coherence tomography. Richdale K, Bullimore MA, Zadnik K. *Ophthalmic Physiol Opt.* 2008 Sep;28(5):441-7.

174. The effects of wearing corrective lenses for presbyopia on distance vision. McGarry MB, Manning TM. *Ophthalmic Physiol Opt.* 2003 Jan;23(1):13-20.

175. Presbyopia correction and the accommodation in reserve. Millodot M, Millodot S. *Ophthalmic Physiol Opt*. 1989 Apr;9(2):126-32.

176. Effect of defocus on visual field measurement. Atchison DA. *Ophthalmic Physiol Opt*. 1987;7(3):259-65.

177. Hexagonal keratotomy for corneal steepening. Grady FJ. *Ophthalmic Surg*. 1988 Sep;19(9):622-3.

178. The NuLens accommodating intraocular lens. Ben-Nun J. *Ophthalmol Clin North Am*. 2006 Mar;19(1):129-34, vii. Review.

179. Sarfarazi dual optic accommodative intraocular lens. Sarfarazi FM. *Ophthalmol Clin North Am*. 2006 Mar;19(1):125-8, vii. Review.

180. Single optic accommodative intraocular lenses. Dick HB, Dell S. *Ophthalmol Clin North Am*. 2006 Mar;19(1):107-24, vi. Review.

181. Presbyopia: perspective on the reality of pseudoaccommodation with LASIK. Telandro AP, Steile J 3rd. *Ophthalmol Clin North Am*. 2006 Mar;19(1):45-69, vi. Review.

182. Keratorefractive approaches to achieving pseudoaccommodation. Trindade F, Pascucci SE. *Ophthalmol Clin North Am*. 2006 Mar;19(1):35-44, vi. Review.

183. Deteriorating vision in the elderly: double stress?. Wahl HW, Heyl Y, Oswald F, Winkler U. *Ophthalmologe*. 1998 Jun;95(6):389-99. German.

184. Accommodating IOLs. Henderson BA. *Ophthalmology*. 2008 Oct;115(10):1850-1.

185. Monovision in LASIK. Braun EH, Lee J, Steinert RF. *Ophthalmology*. 2008 Jul, 115(7):1196-202. Epub 2007 Dec 3.

186. Clear lens extraction with multifocal apodized diffractive intraocular lens implantation. Fernández-Vega L, Alfonso JF, Rodriguez PP, Montés-Micó R. *Ophthalmology*. 2007 Aug;114(8):1491-8. Epub 2007 Mar 13.

187. LASIK in the presbyopic age group: safety, efficacy, and predictability in 40- to 69-year-old patients. Ghanem RC, de la Cruz J, Tobaigy FM, Ang LP, Azar DT. *Ophthalmology*. 2007 Jul;114(7):1303-10. Epub 2007 Mar 26.

188. Presbyopia after keratectomy. Abraham LM, Kuriakose T. *Ophthalmology*. 2007 Apr;114(4):825, author reply 825.

189. Evidence for delayed presbyopia after photorefractive keratectomy for myopia. Artola A, Patel S, Schimchak P, Ayala MJ, Ruiz-Moreno JM, Alió JL. *Ophthalmology*. 2006 May;113(5):735-41.el.

190. Contact lens correction of presbyopia. Morgan PB, Efron N. *Cont Lens Anterior Eye*. 2009 Aug;32(4):191-2. Epub 2009 Jun 16.

191. Iris-fixated anterior chamber phakic intraocular lens for myopia moves posteriorly with mydriasis. Cruysberg LP, Doors M, Berendschot TT, De Brabander J, Webers CA, Nuijts RM. *J Refract Surg*. 2009 Apr;25(4):394-6.

192. Myopia progression in children wearing spectacles vs. switching to contact lenses. Marsh-Tootle WL, Dong LM, Hyman L, Gwiazda J, Weise KK, Dias L, Fernp KD, The COMET Group. *Optom Vis Sci*. 2009 May 7.

193. Short-term adaptive modification of dynamic ocular accommodation. Bharadwaj SR, Vedamurthy I, Schor CM. *Invest Ophthalmol Vis Sci*. 2009 Jul;50(7):3520-8. Epub 2009 Feb 28.

194. LASIK and PRK in refractive accommodative esotropia: a retrospective study on 20 adolescent and adult patients. Magli A, Iovine A, Gagliardi V, Fimiani F, Nucci P. *Eur J Ophthalmol*. 2009 Mar-Apr;19(2):188-95.

195. The pseudoaccommodative cornea multifocal ablation with a center-distance pattern: a review.

Telandro A. *J Refract Surg.* 2009 Jan;25(1 Suppl):S156-9. Review.

196. Pseudoaccommodative cornea treatment using the NIDEK EC-5000 CXIII excimer laser in myopic and hyperopic presbyopes. Uy E,Go R. *J Refract Surg.* 2009 Jan;25(1 Suppl):S148-55.

197. Accommodative lag by autorefraction and two dynamic retinoscopy methods. Correction of Myopia Evaluation Trial 2 Study Group for the Pediatric Eye Disease Investigator Group, Manny RE, Chandler DL, Scheiman MM, Gwiazda JE, Cotter SA, Everett DF, Holmes JM, Hyman LG, Kulp MT, Lyon DW, Marsh-Tootle W, Matta N, Melia BM, Norton TT, Repka MX, Silbert DI, Weissberg EM. *Optom Vis Sci.* 2009 Mar;86(3):233-43.

198. The effect of altering spherical aberration on the static accommodative response. Theagarayan B, Radhakrishnan H, Allen PM, Calver RI, Rae SM, O'Leary DJ. *Ophthalmic Physiol Opt.* 2009 Jan;29(1):65-71.

199. Anticholinergic esotropia. Anderson JM, Brodsky MC. *J Neuroophthalmol.* 2008 Dec;28(4):359-60.

200. Visual field does not affect steady-state accommodative response and near-work induced transient myopia. Yao P, Yang S, Jiang BC. *Vision Res.* 2009 Feb;49(4):490-7. Epub 2009 Jan 10.

201. Initial report of IOL-induced accommodation. Osher RH. *J Cataract Refract Surg.* 2008 Dec;34(12):2009, author reply 2009.

202. Multifocal IOL technology: a successful step on the journey toward presbyopia treatment. Kohnen T. *J Cataract Refract Surg.* 2008 Dec;34(12):2005.

203. Repeatability intraexaminer and agreement in amplitude of accommodation measurements. Antona B, Barra F, Barrio A, Gonzalez E, Sanchez I. *Graefes Arch Clin Exp Ophthalmol.* 2009 Jan;247(1):121-7. Epub 2008 Sep 13.

204. Spherical aberration and depth of focus. Beiko G. *Ophthalmology.* 2008 Sep;115(9):1641, author reply 1641-2.

205. SOP et l'ophtalmologie autrement. Gilg AN, Aillagon-Bourguet. *Ophtalmologie Autrement.* 2008 Sep;1:4-9.

Ouvrages

1. Bouhanna L, *et al. Vade-Mecum d'Ophtalmologie vétérinaire* 2nd edition, edition Med'Com. 2004.

2. Barthelemy B, Thiebault T. *Contactologie,* EMInter Tee & Doc, Lavoisier. 2004.

3. Daniel M Albert, Joan W Miller, Dimitri T Azar, Barbara A Biodi. *Albert & Jakobiec's Principles & Practice on Ophthalmology,* 3rd edition, Saunders. 2008.

4. Tasman, William, Jaeger, Edward A. *Duane's Ophthalmology,* Lippincott Williams & Wilkins (LWW). 2009.

5. Kovarski C Coord. *L'opticien-lunetier,* 2nd edition, Tec & Doc, Lavoisier. 2009.

Index

Page numbers followed by *f* refer to figure and *t* refer to table